# CAUSES OF OBESITY

## "A Comprehensive Exploration"

Christopher K. Fontaine

**Copyright** ©2024 Christopher K. Fontaine



ISBN: 9798878885010

# CONTENTS


Copyright ..................................................................2

INTRODUCTION:.........................................................6

CHAPTER 1: DEFINITION OF OBESITY.........................8

❖ Growing Global Concern:....................................10

❖ Importance of Understanding the Causes: ...................14

CHAPTER 2: GENETIC FACTORS...................................19

❖ Family History and Its Impact on Obesity Risk:...............28

❖ Genetic Conditions Contributing to Weight Gain: .........32

CHAPTER 3: ENVIRONMENTAL FACTORS:......................38

❖ Influence of the Obesogenic Environment: ...................44

❖ Availability and Accessibility of High-Calorie Foods:......50

❖ Sedentary Lifestyle and Lack of Physical Activity:..........55

CHAPTER 4: BEHAVIORAL FACTORS...............................62

❖ Dietary Habits and Choices:....................................67

1. Consumption of high-calorie, low-nutrient foods..........73

2. Overeating and portion sizes ................................78

❖ Physical activity....................................................84

1. Sedentary Lifestyle and Its Consequences:.................91

2. Lack of Regular Exercise:.......................................97

CHAPTER 5: SOCIOECONOMIC FACTORS ......................103

❖ Economic Disparities and Their Impact on Diet:..........109

❖ Access to Health Care and Obesity Prevention:...........116

# Causes of Obesity


❖    Education and Awareness Regarding Healthy Lifestyle Choices:................................................................123

CHAPTER 6: PSYCHOLOGICAL FACTORS....................................131

❖    Emotional Eating and Its Connection to Obesity: ........137

❖    Stress and Its Influence on Eating Behaviors: .............144

❖    Mental Health Issues Contributing to Weight Gain: ....151

CHAPTER 7: MEDICAL CONDITIONS .........................................158

❖    Hormonal Imbalances Affecting Metabolism: .............165

❖    Medications with Potential Side Effects of Weight Gain: 172

❖    Impact of Certain Medical Conditions on Obesity Risk: 177

CHAPTER 8: CULTURAL AND SOCIAL INFLUENCES ...................185

❖    Cultural Norms and Attitudes Towards Body Image:...192

❖    Social Acceptance of Unhealthy Behaviors:................199

❖    Peer Pressure and Its Role in Shaping Lifestyle Choices: 206

CHAPTER 9: CHILDHOOD AND EARLY-LIFE INFLUENCES..........212

❖    Impact of Early Feeding Practices on Obesity Risk: .....219

❖    Childhood Obesity and Its Long-Term Consequences: 225

❖    Parental Influence on Children's Eating Habits and Physical Activity: ...........................................................231

CHAPTER 10: PREVENTION AND INTERVENTION STRATEGIES FOR CHILDHOOD OBESITY ....................................................239

❖    Importance of a Multidimensional Approach in Addressing Childhood Obesity:........................................246

# Causes of Obesity


❖ Public Health Initiatives in Addressing Childhood Obesity:....................................................................254

❖ Individual Responsibility and Lifestyle Modifications in Addressing Childhood Obesity:............................................261

CHAPTER 11: CONCLUSION.................................................269

❖ Recap of Major Causes of Obesity: ...........................272

❖ Call to Action for Addressing the Obesity Epidemic: ...277

❖ Importance of Ongoing Research and Education in Addressing Obesity: ..........................................................285

# INTRODUCTION:

Obesity, a pervasive and escalating health concern, has become a global challenge affecting millions of individuals worldwide. Defined by an excessive accumulation of body fat, obesity poses significant risks to both physical and mental well-being. In recent years, the prevalence of obesity has surged, necessitating a profound understanding of its multifaceted causes. This introduction aims to explore the intricate web of factors contributing to obesity, delving into genetic predispositions, environmental influences, behavioral patterns, socioeconomic disparities, psychological aspects, medical conditions, and cultural influences. By unraveling these interconnected elements, we can gain valuable insights into the complexity of obesity and lay the foundation for effective prevention and intervention strategies. As we embark on this exploration, it becomes evident that addressing obesity requires a holistic approach, encompassing individual choices, societal structures, and global initiatives. Let us navigate through the labyrinth of causes, seeking to comprehend the root of this global health crisis and pave the way towards a healthier future

# CHAPTER 1: DEFINITION OF OBESITY

Obesity, a term derived from the Latin word "obesus," meaning "having eaten until fat," is a medical condition characterized by the excessive accumulation of body fat to the extent that it may have adverse effects on health. It is more than just a cosmetic concern; obesity is recognized as a complex and chronic health issue that significantly increases the risk of various other medical conditions.

The Body Mass Index (BMI) is a commonly used metric to define obesity. BMI is calculated by dividing a person's weight in kilograms by the square of their height in meters. According to the World Health Organization (WHO), a BMI of 30 or higher is indicative of obesity. However, it's essential to note that BMI has its limitations, as it doesn't differentiate between muscle and fat or consider the distribution of fat in the body.

Obesity is often categorized into different classes based on BMI:

1. Class 1 (Moderate Obesity): BMI between 30 and 34.9

2. Class 2 (Severe Obesity): BMI between 35 and 39.9

3. Class 3 (Very Severe or Morbid Obesity): BMI of 40 and above

Apart from BMI, other factors, such as waist circumference and waist-to-hip ratio, are also considered when assessing the health implications of excess body fat. These measurements provide a more nuanced understanding of fat distribution, with abdominal fat (visceral fat) being particularly associated with increased health risks.

Obesity is not solely a cosmetic concern; it has profound implications for one's health. It is linked to a higher risk of developing various chronic conditions, including heart disease, type 2 diabetes, certain cancers, and musculoskeletal disorders. Additionally, obesity can impact mental health, contributing to issues like depression and reduced quality of life.

Understanding the definition of obesity is crucial in our exploration of its causes, as it lays the groundwork for comprehending the magnitude and severity of this global health challenge.

## ❖ Growing Global Concern:

In recent decades, obesity has emerged as a burgeoning global concern, transcending geographical boundaries and affecting diverse populations. The prevalence of obesity has reached alarming proportions, prompting health organizations, policymakers, and communities to recognize it as a multifaceted challenge that extends beyond individual health to societal well-being and economic stability.

1. Epidemiological Shifts: The epidemiological landscape has undergone a transformative shift, with obesity transitioning from a concern primarily in high-income countries to a pervasive issue affecting people across all income levels and regions. Developing nations, in particular, are witnessing a rapid increase in obesity rates, further emphasizing the global nature of this health crisis.

2. Health and Economic Implications: The consequences of obesity extend far beyond individual health. The economic burden associated with treating obesity-related conditions, such as diabetes, cardiovascular diseases, and certain

cancers, places a substantial strain on healthcare systems globally. The intersection of health and economic implications underscores the urgency of addressing obesity as a priority public health issue.

3.     Lifestyle Changes: Societal changes in lifestyle, including shifts in dietary patterns and sedentary behaviors, have contributed to the rise in obesity. Globalization, urbanization, and the availability of processed, high-calorie foods have altered traditional eating habits, fostering an environment conducive to weight gain.

4.     Nutritional Transition: The nutritional transition, characterized by a shift from traditional, locally sourced diets to diets high in refined sugars, saturated fats, and processed foods, has played a pivotal role in the obesity epidemic. This transition is often linked to increased urbanization and changes

in food production and distribution systems.

5.    Technological Advances: Advances in technology have led to a reduction in physical activity levels. Sedentary occupations, increased screen time, and a decline in active transportation contribute to a more sedentary lifestyle, further exacerbating the obesity epidemic.

6.    Social Determinants: Social determinants, such as income inequality, education levels, and access to healthcare, contribute significantly to obesity disparities. Individuals with limited resources may face barriers to adopting healthy lifestyles, creating a cycle of disadvantage.

7.    Childhood Obesity: The prevalence of childhood obesity has reached alarming levels globally. Early exposure to unhealthy food choices, coupled with

limited opportunities for physical activity, sets the stage for a lifelong struggle with weight-related issues.

Recognizing obesity as a growing global concern is a crucial step in addressing the root causes and implementing effective strategies for prevention and intervention. The interconnectedness of factors contributing to obesity necessitates a collaborative, interdisciplinary approach to create sustainable solutions that promote health and well-being on a global scale.

## ❖ Importance of Understanding the Causes:

Comprehending the myriad causes of obesity is pivotal for several compelling reasons, ranging from individual well-being to broader public health and socioeconomic considerations. The significance of understanding these causes lies in the ability to develop targeted interventions, implement preventive measures, and cultivate a comprehensive approach to tackle the obesity epidemic.

1. Tailored Interventions: Understanding the diverse causes of obesity allows for the development of tailored interventions that address specific contributing factors. Individuals may have unique combinations of genetic predispositions, environmental exposures, and behavioral patterns, necessitating personalized approaches for effective prevention and treatment.

2. Public Health Strategies: Identifying the root causes of obesity is crucial for formulating effective public health strategies. By addressing the multifaceted nature of the issue, policymakers can implement evidence-based interventions that encompass education, healthcare access, and

community programs. This, in turn, can help mitigate the societal burden of obesity-related diseases.

3.    Prevention Efforts: Prevention is key to curbing the obesity epidemic. Knowledge of the causes enables the design of preventive measures that target risk factors at various levels, from individual behaviors to societal and environmental influences. These efforts can promote healthier lifestyles and reduce the incidence of obesity-related conditions.

4.    Healthcare Planning and Resource Allocation: Understanding the causes of obesity aids in healthcare planning and resource allocation. With insights into the factors contributing to obesity, healthcare systems can allocate resources efficiently, focusing on early intervention, education, and support for affected individuals.

5.    Individual Empowerment: Knowledge empowers individuals to make informed choices about their health. Understanding the causes of obesity enables individuals to recognize risk factors in their lives, make lifestyle adjustments, and seek appropriate support. This empowerment fosters a sense of agency and responsibility for one's well-being.

6.    Addressing Disparities: Recognizing the social determinants of obesity allows for targeted efforts to address health disparities. Understanding how factors such as income, education, and access to healthcare contribute to obesity helps formulate strategies that aim to reduce disparities and promote health equity.

7.    Long-Term Impact: A comprehensive understanding of the causes of obesity contributes to long-term solutions. By addressing root

causes rather than just symptoms, interventions can have a lasting impact on reducing obesity rates and preventing associated health conditions.

8.      Interdisciplinary Collaboration: Obesity is a complex issue that requires collaboration across various disciplines, including healthcare, nutrition, psychology, urban planning, and policy. Understanding the diverse causes facilitates interdisciplinary collaboration, fostering a holistic and integrated approach to combating obesity.

In conclusion, delving into the causes of obesity is not only academically valuable but also holds immense practical importance. It serves as the foundation for targeted interventions, informed decision-making at individual and societal levels, and the development of sustainable strategies to address this global health challenge.

# CHAPTER 2: GENETIC FACTORS

Genetic factors play a substantial role in shaping an individual's susceptibility to obesity. While lifestyle choices and environmental influences contribute significantly to weight management, understanding the genetic underpinnings provides crucial insights into why certain individuals may be predisposed to obesity.

1.    Genetic Predisposition:

•    Inherited Traits: The heritability of obesity is evident in familial clustering and the transmission of certain physical and metabolic traits from parents to offspring. Genetic factors contribute to approximately 40-70% of the variability in body weight.

•    Polygenic Nature: Obesity is polygenic, involving the interplay of multiple genes. Numerous genetic variants, each with a modest effect, collectively contribute to an individual's predisposition to weight gain.

2.    Leptin and Ghrelin Regulation:

•    Leptin Resistance: Leptin is a hormone that regulates appetite and energy expenditure. Genetic factors can lead to leptin resistance, where the body fails to respond appropriately to this satiety signal, potentially resulting in overeating.

•    Ghrelin Sensitivity: Genetic variations can also influence the sensitivity to ghrelin, a hormone that stimulates appetite. Altered ghrelin response may contribute to increased hunger and, consequently, weight gain.

3.    Metabolic Rate and Energy Expenditure:

•    Basal Metabolic Rate (BMR): Genetic factors contribute to individual variations in BMR, influencing the number of calories burned at rest. Those with a lower BMR may find it more challenging to maintain a healthy weight.

•	Energy Efficiency: Genetic variations can affect energy efficiency, influencing how efficiently the body converts food into energy or stores it as fat.

4.	Fat Storage and Distribution:

•	Adipogenesis Genes: Genetic factors influence adipogenesis, the process of fat cell development. Variations in genes related to adipogenesis can impact the number and size of fat cells, contributing to obesity.

•	Distribution Patterns: Genes play a role in determining where the body stores fat. Apple-shaped (central) or pear-shaped (peripheral) fat distribution can have different implications for health.

5.    Neurotransmitter and Hormone Regulation:

•    Dopamine and Serotonin Pathways: Genetic variations in dopamine and serotonin pathways may influence reward-seeking behaviors and emotional eating, contributing to overconsumption of high-calorie foods.

•    Insulin Sensitivity: Genetic factors can affect insulin sensitivity, impacting how the body regulates blood sugar. Insulin resistance may lead to increased fat storage and weight gain.

6.    Rare Genetic Syndromes:

•    Monogenic Obesity Syndromes: In rare cases, single gene mutations can lead to severe obesity. Examples include Prader-Willi syndrome and Bardet-Biedl syndrome, highlighting the diverse genetic factors influencing body weight.

Understanding the genetic factors associated with obesity is pivotal not only for elucidating individual susceptibility but also for informing personalized approaches to weight management. While genetic predisposition sets the stage, the interplay with environmental factors remains a crucial aspect of the obesity puzzle. This knowledge underscores the importance of holistic strategies that address both genetic and lifestyle influences for effective obesity prevention and management.

## ❖ Role of Genetics in Predisposing Individuals to Obesity:

Genetic factors significantly contribute to an individual's predisposition to obesity, shaping various aspects of metabolism, appetite regulation, and fat storage.

Understanding the intricate role of genetics in obesity provides valuable insights into why certain individuals may be more susceptible to weight gain, laying the groundwork for personalized interventions and preventative measures.

1.    Heritability of Obesity:

•    Familial Clustering: Observations of obesity running in families highlight the heritability of this condition. Individuals with obese parents are more likely to be obese themselves, pointing to a genetic component in weight regulation.

•    Twin Studies: Studies on identical and non-identical twins reveal a higher concordance of obesity in identical twins, supporting the genetic influence on body weight.

2.    Polygenic Nature:

- Multiple Genetic Variants: Obesity is not determined by a single gene but rather by the cumulative effects of multiple genetic variants. The polygenic nature of obesity involves interactions among various genes, each contributing in a modest manner to the overall risk.

- Genome-Wide Association Studies (GWAS): GWAS have identified numerous genetic loci associated with obesity, shedding light on the complex genetic architecture of this condition.

3. Hormonal Regulation:

- Leptin and Ghrelin Genes: Genetic variations in genes related to leptin and ghrelin, hormones crucial for appetite regulation, can impact an individual's susceptibility to overeating and weight gain.

- Insulin Signaling Pathway: Genetic factors influence the insulin signaling pathway, affecting how the body utilizes glucose and stores fat. Altered insulin sensitivity may contribute to obesity.

4.    Metabolic Rate:

•    Genetic Influence on BMR: Basal Metabolic Rate (BMR), the energy expended at rest, is influenced by genetic factors. Individuals with a genetically determined lower BMR may find it challenging to maintain a healthy weight.

•    Energy Expenditure: Genetic variations can affect energy expenditure during physical activity, influencing how efficiently the body burns calories.

5.    Fat Storage and Distribution:

•    Adiposity Genes: Genes associated with adipogenesis and fat cell development impact the body's ability to store and regulate fat. Variations in these genes can contribute to obesity.

•	Body Fat Distribution Genes: Genetic factors influence where the body tends to store fat. Some individuals may have a genetic predisposition for central (abdominal) obesity, which is associated with higher health risks.

6.	Neurotransmitter Pathways:

•	Dopamine and Serotonin Receptor Genes: Genetic variations in dopamine and serotonin receptors may influence reward-seeking behaviors and emotional eating, contributing to overconsumption of calories.

Understanding the role of genetics in obesity is essential for recognizing that individuals have varying degrees of genetic susceptibility. While genetics may set the stage for weight regulation, environmental factors, lifestyle choices, and cultural influences also play pivotal roles. This knowledge emphasizes the importance of personalized strategies that consider both genetic and environmental factors for effective obesity prevention and management.

## ❖ Family History and Its Impact on Obesity Risk:

The influence of family history on obesity risk is a significant aspect of understanding the genetic predisposition to this complex condition. Families often share not only genetic traits but also lifestyle habits and environmental factors, contributing to the interplay between genetics and environment in the development of obesity.

1.    Genetic Inheritance:

•    Hereditary Patterns: Individuals with a family history of obesity are more likely to inherit genetic factors that predispose them to weight gain. The transmission of genetic variants associated with metabolism, appetite regulation, and fat storage contributes to the familial clustering of obesity.

•	Monogenic Obesity Syndromes: Rare but severe forms of obesity may result from specific genetic mutations inherited within families, emphasizing the direct genetic contribution to excessive weight.

2.	Shared Environment:

•	Common Lifestyle Habits: Families often share common lifestyle habits, including dietary patterns and physical activity levels. These shared behaviors can contribute to similarities in body weight among family members.

•	Early Life Influences: Childhood experiences within a family, such as dietary habits learned at home and the importance placed on physical activity, can influence long-term health behaviors and contribute to obesity risk.

3.    Epigenetic Factors:

•    Epigenetic Modifications: Beyond genetic inheritance, epigenetic factors play a role in regulating gene expression. Environmental influences within a family, such as nutrition during pregnancy and early childhood, can lead to epigenetic modifications that impact an individual's susceptibility to obesity.

4.    Cultural and Dietary Practices:

•    Cultural Norms: Families often share cultural norms related to food choices, meal patterns, and the significance of certain foods. Cultural influences can shape dietary practices that contribute to obesity risk.

•    Dietary Environment at Home: The availability of high-calorie, processed foods at home and family meal dynamics influence individual dietary choices and can contribute to weight-related issues.

5.  Social Support and Influence:

•  Social Dynamics: The level of social support within a family can influence an individual's ability to adopt and maintain healthy lifestyle habits. Supportive family environments may facilitate weight management efforts, while unsupportive environments can pose challenges.

•  Role Modeling: Family members often serve as role models for behaviors related to eating and physical activity. Observing unhealthy habits or sedentary lifestyles within the family can impact an individual's own choices.

6.  Psychosocial Factors:

•  Stress and Coping Mechanisms: Family environments can contribute to psychosocial factors, such as stress levels and coping mechanisms. Emotional eating often learned or reinforced within families, can be a contributing factor to obesity.

Understanding the impact of family history on obesity risk emphasizes the need for a holistic approach to address both genetic and environmental factors. While genetic predisposition plays a role, modifying shared lifestyle habits, promoting healthy environments within families, and fostering individual resilience are essential components of effective obesity prevention and intervention strategies.

❖ **Genetic Conditions Contributing to Weight Gain:**

Certain genetic conditions can directly contribute to weight gain by affecting various aspects of metabolism, appetite regulation, and energy expenditure. These conditions highlight the diverse ways in which genetic factors can influence an individual's susceptibility to obesity.

1.    Prader-Willi Syndrome (PWS):

•    Genetic Basis: PWS is a rare genetic disorder caused by the loss of function of specific genes on chromosome 15. This genetic abnormality leads to a range of physical, cognitive, and behavioral challenges.

•    Hyperphagia: Individuals with PWS often experience an insatiable appetite (hyperphagia), leading to excessive eating. This behavioral aspect, combined with reduced energy expenditure, contributes to significant weight gain.

2.    Bardet-Biedl Syndrome (BBS):

• Genetic Basis: BBS is a rare genetic disorder characterized by various features, including obesity, retinal degeneration, and kidney abnormalities. It results from mutations in multiple genes.

• Leptin and Ghrelin Dysregulation: Genetic factors associated with BBS can disrupt the normal regulation of hormones like leptin and ghrelin, impacting appetite control and leading to obesity.

3. Leptin Receptor Deficiency:

• Genetic Mutation: Mutations in the gene coding for the leptin receptor can result in a condition where the body does not respond adequately to the appetite-regulating hormone leptin.

• Hyperphagia and Reduced Energy Expenditure: Individuals with leptin receptor deficiency may experience constant hunger (hyperphagia) and reduced energy expenditure, contributing to significant weight gain.

4.     Melanocortin-4 Receptor (MC4R) Deficiency:

•     Genetic Mutation: MC4R is involved in appetite regulation, and mutations in the gene can lead to a deficiency in the receptor.

•     Increased Appetite and Reduced Satiety: Individuals with MC4R deficiency may have an increased appetite and reduced satiety, making it challenging to regulate food intake and resulting in weight gain.

5.     Ahlstrom Syndrome:

•     Genetic Basis: Alström syndrome is a rare genetic disorder caused by mutations in the ALMS1 gene. It affects various organs, including the heart, liver, and kidneys.

• Obesity and Insulin Resistance: Alström syndrome is often associated with early-onset obesity and insulin resistance, contributing to metabolic complications.

6. Cohen Syndrome:

• Genetic Basis: Cohen syndrome is a genetic disorder caused by mutations in the VPS13B gene. It affects various systems, leading to intellectual disabilities, facial abnormalities, and obesity.

• Hyperphagia and Obesity: Individuals with Cohen syndrome may exhibit hyperphagia, leading to overeating and obesity as a prominent feature of the condition.

7. Down Syndrome:

• Genetic Basis: Down syndrome results from the presence of an extra copy of chromosome 21. While not all individuals with Down syndrome experience obesity, a higher prevalence of overweight and obesity has been observed.

• Metabolic Factors: Metabolic factors related to Down syndrome, such as reduced muscle tone and lower metabolic rate, may contribute to weight gain.

Understanding these genetic conditions contributing to weight gain provides insights into the intricate mechanisms regulating body weight. While these conditions are rare, they underscore the importance of genetic factors in shaping metabolic pathways and appetite regulation. Additionally, research on these conditions contributes to broader knowledge about the genetic basis of obesity and potential targets for therapeutic interventions.

## CHAPTER 3: ENVIRONMENTAL FACTORS:

Environmental factors play a pivotal role in shaping lifestyles, dietary choices, and physical activity patterns, all of which contribute significantly to the global obesity epidemic. Understanding how the environment influences individuals is crucial for developing effective interventions and public health strategies to address and prevent obesity.

1.    Obesogenic Environment:

•    Definition: The term "obesogenic environment" refers to an environment that promotes behaviors leading to weight gain and obesity. This includes factors such as the availability of high-calorie, low-nutrient foods, sedentary lifestyles, and limited opportunities for physical activity.

•      Processed Foods: The ready availability of processed, energy-dense foods high in sugars and fats contributes to unhealthy eating habits and weight gain.

•      Sedentary Lifestyle: Modern environments often encourage sedentary behaviors, with increased screen time, desk jobs, and reliance on motorized transportation, all contributing to reduced physical activity.

2.      Food Accessibility and Availability:

•      Food Deserts: Certain neighborhoods may lack access to fresh, nutritious foods, creating food deserts where residents rely on convenience stores with limited healthy options. This can contribute to poor dietary choices and obesity.

•      Fast Food Culture: The prevalence of fast-food establishments and the ease of access to high-calorie, low-nutrient foods contribute to unhealthy eating patterns and weight gain.

3.	Built Environment:

•	Urban Design: The design of urban spaces influences physical activity levels. Walkable neighborhoods, accessible parks, and bike-friendly infrastructure encourage active lifestyles and can contribute to weight management.

•	Transportation Infrastructure: Cities with extensive public transportation and pedestrian-friendly infrastructure promote active commuting, reducing reliance on sedentary modes of transportation.

4.	Social and Cultural Influences:

•	Social Norms: Cultural attitudes and social norms surrounding body image, eating habits, and physical activity influence individual behaviors.

Pressure to conform to certain body ideals may contribute to unhealthy weight control practices.

•	Social Support Systems: The presence or absence of supportive social networks can impact an individual's ability to maintain a healthy lifestyle. Positive social influences encourage healthy behaviors, while negative influences may hinder them.

5.	Advertising and Marketing:

•	Food Advertising: The pervasive marketing of unhealthy foods, especially to children, can influence dietary preferences and contribute to the consumption of high-calorie, low-nutrient products.

•	Sedentary Entertainment: The promotion of sedentary entertainment options, such as video games and screen-based activities, can contribute to a more sedentary lifestyle, especially among children and adolescents.

6.    Workplace Environment:

•    Occupational Sedentary Behavior: Sedentary occupations contribute to a lack of physical activity during working hours. Workplaces that encourage movement, standing desks, and physical activity breaks can counteract these effects.

•    Access to Healthy Options: The availability of healthy food options in workplace cafeterias and vending machines can influence dietary choices among employees.

7.    Economic Disparities:

•    Access to Healthy Foods: Economic disparities can impact access to fresh, nutritious foods. Individuals with lower incomes may face challenges affording healthier options, leading to reliance on more affordable but less nutritious alternatives.

•      Recreation Opportunities: Wealthier communities often have better access to recreational facilities, parks, and fitness programs, providing more opportunities for physical activity.

8.      Educational and Informational Factors:

•      Nutrition Education: The level of nutrition education and awareness in communities can influence dietary choices. Lack of knowledge about healthy eating may contribute to the consumption of energy-dense, nutrient-poor foods.

•      Health Literacy: Limited health literacy can hinder individuals' ability to understand and act upon health information, impacting their ability to make informed choices about diet and lifestyle.

Understanding the environmental factors contributing to obesity is essential for developing targeted interventions and policies that promote healthier behaviors. Addressing these factors requires a multifaceted approach involving community planning, public health initiatives, and education to create environments that support and encourage healthy lifestyles.

❖ **Influence of the Obesogenic Environment:**

The obesogenic environment, characterized by factors that encourage unhealthy dietary habits and sedentary lifestyles, significantly contributes to the rising global prevalence of obesity. This environment plays a pivotal role in shaping individual behaviors, making it essential to explore its various influences on weight gain.

1.   Food Environment:

•   High-Calorie, Low-Nutrient Foods: The obesogenic environment is characterized by the ready availability of energy-dense, nutrient-poor foods. Fast food outlets, convenience stores, and vending machines often offer easily accessible options that are high in sugars, fats, and calories.

•   Large Portion Sizes: Restaurants and food establishments often promote larger portion sizes, contributing to overconsumption of calories in a single sitting.

2.   Marketing and Advertising:

•   Promotion of Unhealthy Foods: Advertising and marketing campaigns often promote unhealthy food choices, especially targeting children and adolescents. The constant exposure to enticing advertisements can influence preferences and drive the consumption of high-calorie products.

•      Food Endorsements: Celebrity endorsements and the association of popular figures with unhealthy food products contribute to the normalization of such choices.

3.      Sedentary Lifestyle Promotion:

•      Screen-Based Entertainment: The prevalence of screen-based entertainment, including television, video games, and social media, encourages sedentary behaviors. Excessive screen time is linked to reduced physical activity and increased snacking.

•      Desk Jobs and Commuting: Occupational settings that require prolonged periods of sitting, coupled with sedentary commuting habits, contribute to an overall decrease in physical activity.

4.     Built Environment:

•     Lack of Walkable Spaces: Urban planning that prioritizes vehicular transportation over walkability contributes to reduced physical activity. Lack of sidewalks, parks, and safe recreational spaces limits opportunities for active living.

•     Limited Access to Green Spaces: Insufficient access to parks and green spaces discourages outdoor activities and exercise, particularly in urban environments.

5.     Social and Cultural Influences:

•     Body Image Standards: Societal pressures and cultural norms around body image can influence behaviors related to weight control. The pursuit of unrealistic body ideals may lead to unhealthy dieting practices or the adoption of extreme weight loss measures.

•      Social Acceptance of Unhealthy Habits: Social acceptance of sedentary behaviors and unhealthy dietary choices within communities can normalize such habits, making it challenging for individuals to adopt healthier lifestyles.

6.     Food Deserts:

•      Limited Access to Healthy Foods: In certain neighborhoods, the lack of grocery stores offering fresh, nutritious foods creates food deserts. Residents may rely on convenience stores with limited healthy options, contributing to poor dietary choices and obesity.

7.     Technological Advances:

•      Automated Transportation: Technological advances in transportation, such as automobiles and ride-sharing services, reduce the need for physical activity in daily routines.

•	Convenience Devices: Labor-saving devices and conveniences, such as elevators and escalators, further reduce incidental physical activity.

8.	Economic Disparities:

•	Affordability of Unhealthy Foods: Economic disparities can impact the affordability of nutritious foods. In lower-income communities, individuals may have limited resources, making cheaper but less nutritious food options more appealing.

•	Access to Recreational Facilities: Wealthier communities often have better access to recreational facilities and fitness programs, creating disparities in opportunities for physical activity.

Understanding the influence of the obesogenic environment is essential for designing interventions that address these environmental factors. Public health initiatives, policy changes, and community-based programs can work towards creating environments that promote healthier choices, making it easier for individuals to adopt and maintain a lifestyle conducive to weight management.

## ❖ Availability and Accessibility of High-Calorie Foods:

The pervasive availability and accessibility of high-calorie foods contribute significantly to the obesogenic environment, influencing dietary choices and contributing to the global obesity epidemic. Various factors contribute to the prevalence of these foods, making them easily obtainable and tempting for individuals, often leading to overconsumption.

1.   Fast Food Chains and Restaurants:

• Widespread Presence: Fast-food chains and restaurants are omnipresent, offering convenient and quick options that are often high in calories, saturated fats, and sugars.

• Large Portions: The practice of offering large portion sizes encourages overeating and contributes to excessive calorie intake.

2. Convenience Stores and Vending Machines:

• 24/7 Access: Convenience stores and vending machines provide round-the-clock access to high-calorie snacks, sugary beverages, and processed foods.

• Impulse Purchases: The placement of high-calorie items at eye level and near checkout counters encourages impulse purchases, contributing to unplanned consumption.

3.    Processed and Packaged Foods:

•    Ubiquity of Processed Foods: Highly processed and packaged foods, often high in added sugars, fats, and salt, line the aisles of grocery stores.

•    Marketing Strategies: Clever marketing strategies, including vibrant packaging and persuasive labeling, attract consumers to these high-calorie options.

4.    Sugar-Sweetened Beverages:

•    Widespread Availability: Sugar-sweetened beverages, including sodas and sweetened juices, are widely available in vending machines, convenience stores, and restaurants.

•    Portion Sizes and Refills: Larger portion sizes and the availability of free refills contribute to excessive consumption of sugary drinks.

5.    Marketing and Advertising:

- Targeted Advertising: Aggressive marketing of high-calorie foods, especially targeting children and adolescents, influences brand preferences and encourages consumption.

- Product Placement: Strategic product placement in stores and promotional campaigns further increase the visibility and desirability of these foods.

6. Food Deserts:

- Limited Access to Fresh Foods: In areas classified as food deserts, where fresh and nutritious food options are scarce, residents may rely on high-calorie, processed foods due to limited choices.

- Impact on Dietary Choices: The lack of access to fresh produce and healthier alternatives influences dietary habits, contributing to the consumption of calorie-dense options.

7.   Online and Delivery Services:

•   Digital Accessibility: The rise of online platforms and food delivery services provides easy access to a wide array of high-calorie foods without requiring physical presence in food establishments.

•   Promotional Deals: Promotional deals and discounts on online food orders may encourage larger orders and frequent consumption of high-calorie options.

8.   School and Workplace Environments:

•   Vending Machines in Schools: Schools often have vending machines offering snacks and beverages that are high in calories and low in nutritional value.

•    Workplace Cafeterias: Workplace cafeterias may prioritize convenience over health, offering calorie-dense options that appeal to taste preferences.

Addressing the availability and accessibility of high-calorie foods is crucial for curbing obesity rates. Interventions may include policy changes, nutritional education, and community initiatives aimed at promoting healthier food environments. By fostering environments that make nutritious choices more accessible, individuals can be empowered to make healthier decisions, contributing to the prevention and management of obesity.

❖ Sedentary Lifestyle and Lack of Physical Activity:

The prevalence of sedentary lifestyles and insufficient physical activity is a significant contributor to the obesogenic environment, playing a central role in the global obesity epidemic. Various societal, technological, and environmental factors contribute to a reduction in physical activity levels, impacting overall health and contributing to weight gain.

1.    Technological Advances:

•    Screen-Based Entertainment: The rise of screen-based entertainment, including television, video games, and digital devices, encourages sedentary behaviors. Excessive screen time often replaces active pursuits.

•    Desk Jobs: The prevalence of sedentary occupations, characterized by prolonged periods of sitting at desks, contributes to reduced daily physical activity.

2.    Transportation Habits:

•      Automobile Dependence: Reliance on automobiles for commuting and transportation reduces opportunities for walking or cycling, contributing to a more sedentary lifestyle.

•      Public Transportation: While public transportation can be a more active alternative, individuals may still experience long periods of sitting during their commutes.

3.     Urban Design and Infrastructure:

•      Lack of Walkable Spaces: Urban planning that prioritizes vehicular traffic over pedestrian-friendly designs limits opportunities for walking. Absence of sidewalks and green spaces discourages outdoor activities.

•      Limited Access to Recreation: Insufficient access to recreational facilities, parks, and fitness centers hinders engagement in physical activities.

4.   Occupational Settings:

•   Sedentary Jobs: Many occupations involve prolonged periods of sitting or require minimal physical exertion. Sedentary jobs contribute to a lack of movement during working hours.

•   Long Work Hours: Lengthy work hours may leave individuals with little time or energy for physical activity outside of their jobs.

5.   Screen Time and Digital Devices:

•   Increased Screen Time: Excessive use of digital devices for work, entertainment, and socializing contributes to a sedentary lifestyle, particularly among children and adolescents.

•   Sedentary Recreation: Video games, streaming services, and social media often promote sedentary recreation, displacing more active forms of leisure.

6.    Cultural and Lifestyle Habits:

•    Shift in Leisure Activities: Changes in cultural and lifestyle habits have shifted leisure activities towards more sedentary options, such as binge-watching television series or spending extended periods on digital devices.

•    Social Gatherings: Socializing often revolves around activities that involve minimal physical activity, such as sitting for meals or gatherings.

7.    Limited Access to Physical Education:

•    Educational Settings: Reduced emphasis on physical education programs in schools limits opportunities for children and adolescents to engage in regular physical activity.

- Homework and Academic Pressure: Increased academic pressure and homework may further limit the time available for physical activities among students.

8. Social and Environmental Influences:

- Social Norms: Societal norms that prioritize convenience and comfort over physical exertion contribute to the acceptance of sedentary behaviors.

- Lack of Role Models: Limited exposure to active role models and the glorification of sedentary lifestyles in media may influence behavior.

Addressing sedentary lifestyles requires a multi-faceted approach involving changes in societal norms, urban planning, workplace policies, and educational practices. Encouraging regular physical activity through community initiatives, promoting active transportation, and integrating movement into daily routines are crucial steps in mitigating the impact of sedentary behaviors on obesity and overall health.

# CHAPTER 4: BEHAVIORAL FACTORS

Behavioral factors play a pivotal role in the development and management of obesity. Individual choices and habits related to diet, physical activity, and lifestyle contribute significantly to weight outcomes. Understanding these behavioral factors is essential for designing effective interventions that empower individuals to make healthier choices.

1. Dietary Choices:

• Food Selection: The types of foods individuals choose to consume greatly influence their calorie intake. Diets high in processed foods, sugars, and saturated fats contribute to excess calorie consumption.

• Portion Control: Overeating, often linked to larger portion sizes and mindless eating, can lead to an imbalance between calorie intake and expenditure.

2.   Eating Habits:

•   Eating Speed: Rapid eating is associated with overeating, as the body may not have enough time to signal fullness. Slow and mindful eating can contribute to better appetite regulation.

•   Emotional Eating: Using food as a coping mechanism for stress, boredom, or emotional distress can lead to excessive calorie intake and weight gain.

3.   Physical Activity Levels:

•   Regular Exercise: The absence of regular physical activity contributes to a sedentary lifestyle, hindering efforts to maintain a healthy weight.

•   Inconsistent Exercise Routine: Lack of consistency in exercise routines can impede long-term weight management efforts.

4.    Sedentary Behaviors:

•    Screen Time: Excessive screen time, whether for work or leisure, is associated with sedentary behaviors and reduced physical activity.

•    Desk-bound Jobs: Occupations that require prolonged periods of sitting contribute to overall sedentary behavior.

5.    Stress Management:

•    Stress Eating: Unhealthy coping mechanisms, such as stress eating or emotional overeating, can contribute to weight gain.

•    Mindfulness and Relaxation: Adopting stress-management techniques, such as mindfulness and relaxation exercises, can positively impact eating behaviors.

6.   Sleep Patterns:

•   Inadequate Sleep: Poor sleep patterns and inadequate sleep duration have been linked to disruptions in hunger-regulating hormones, leading to increased appetite and cravings.

•   Late-Night Eating: Irregular sleep patterns may contribute to late-night snacking and unhealthy eating habits.

7.   Social and Environmental Influences:

•   Social Support: Supportive social networks and positive peer influences can enhance healthy behaviors, including dietary choices and physical activity.

•   Food Environment: Access to healthy foods and the presence of high-calorie options in the immediate environment influence dietary decisions.

8.   Self-Monitoring:

• Awareness of Habits: Regular self-monitoring of dietary habits, physical activity levels, and weight can enhance awareness and promote accountability.

• Goal Setting: Establishing realistic and achievable goals for diet and exercise helps individuals stay focused and motivated.

9. Cultural and Socioeconomic Factors:

• Cultural Influences: Cultural norms related to food preferences, eating habits, and body image play a role in shaping individual behaviors.

• Socioeconomic Status: Economic factors can impact access to healthy foods, recreational facilities, and opportunities for physical activity.

10. Health Literacy:

• Understanding Nutrition: A lack of understanding about nutrition and healthy lifestyle choices can contribute to poor dietary decisions.

•       Interpreting Food Labels: Improving health literacy, particularly in interpreting food labels, empowers individuals to make informed choices about their diet.

Understanding and addressing these behavioral factors require a comprehensive and individualized approach. Behavioral interventions, lifestyle coaching, and education play essential roles in promoting healthier choices and sustainable habits for long-term weight management. Empowering individuals to make positive changes in their behaviors is key to combating obesity on both individual and societal levels.

❖ **Dietary Habits and Choices:**
Dietary habits and choices are pivotal behavioral factors influencing body

weight and overall health. The types of foods individuals select, their portion sizes, and the frequency of certain dietary behaviors contribute significantly to the complex landscape of obesity. Understanding these aspects is crucial for promoting healthier eating habits and preventing excessive weight gain.

1.    Food Selection:

•    Nutrient-Dense Choices: Opting for nutrient-dense foods, such as fruits, vegetables, whole grains, and lean proteins, contributes to a balanced and healthful diet.

•    Processed and Sugary Foods: Regular consumption of processed foods, high in sugars and saturated fats, can contribute to excessive calorie intake and weight gain.

2.    Portion Control:

• Balanced Serving Sizes: Practicing portion control helps individuals manage their calorie intake and prevents overeating. Being mindful of serving sizes is essential for weight management.

• Mindful Eating: Adopting mindful eating practices, such as paying attention to hunger and fullness cues, promotes healthier portion control.

3. Meal Timing:

• Regular Meals: Establishing regular meal patterns helps maintain stable energy levels and prevents excessive snacking between meals.

• Late-Night Eating: Consuming large meals or snacks late at night may disrupt the body's natural circadian rhythms and contribute to weight gain.

4. Hydration Habits:

•      Water Consumption: Choosing water as the primary beverage over sugary drinks helps reduce overall calorie intake and supports hydration.

•      Alcohol Consumption: Moderating alcohol intake is essential, as alcoholic beverages contribute additional calories and may lead to poor food choices.

5.      Food Preparation Methods:

•      Cooking Methods: Choosing healthier cooking methods, such as grilling, baking, or steaming, over frying, contributes to lower calorie content in meals.

•      Limiting Added Fats and Sauces: Minimizing the use of added fats, oils, and high-calorie sauces supports healthier food preparation.

6.      Snacking Patterns:

•      Healthy Snack Choices: Opting for nutritious snacks, such as fruits, vegetables, or nuts, supports weight management between meals.

• Mindful Snacking: Being mindful of portion sizes during snacks helps prevent excessive calorie consumption throughout the day.

7. Cultural and Social Influences:

• Traditional Eating Patterns: Cultural influences play a role in shaping dietary habits. Maintaining traditional eating patterns that emphasize whole foods can contribute to a balanced diet.

• Social Eating: Being aware of social influences on eating behaviors helps individuals make conscious choices in various social settings.

8. Emotional Eating:

• Coping Mechanisms: Recognizing emotional eating patterns and finding alternative coping mechanisms for stress, boredom, or emotions reduces reliance on food for emotional support.

•    Mindful Consumption: Practicing mindful eating during emotional situations helps foster a healthier relationship with food.

9.    Label Reading and Nutrition Awareness:

•    Interpreting Food Labels: Developing the ability to interpret food labels empowers individuals to make informed choices about the nutritional content of packaged foods.

•    Nutritional Education: Enhancing nutritional literacy and understanding the impact of food choices on health promotes healthier dietary decisions.

10.    Goal Setting and Planning:

•    Setting Dietary Goals: Establishing realistic dietary goals helps individuals stay focused on making positive changes.

•	Meal Planning: Planning meals in advance supports healthier food choices and prevents reliance on convenient but less nutritious options.

Encouraging healthier dietary habits involves a combination of education, behavioral interventions, and environmental supports. Empowering individuals to make informed and mindful choices about their diet is essential for long-term weight management and overall well-being.

## 1. Consumption of high-calorie, low-nutrient foods

The consumption of high-calorie, low-nutrient foods is a significant behavioral factor that contributes to the development and exacerbation of obesity. This dietary habit involves regularly choosing foods that are energy-dense but provide little nutritional value. Understanding the impact of this behavior on overall health is crucial for promoting better food choices and preventing weight-related issues. Several factors contribute to the prevalence of consuming such foods:

1.    Processed Foods:

•    Energy Density: Many processed foods, such as snacks, sweets, and fast-food items, are characterized by high energy density due to added sugars, fats, and refined carbohydrates.

•    Low Nutrient Content: Despite their calorie density, these foods often lack essential nutrients like vitamins, minerals, and fiber, leading to empty calorie consumption.

2.    Fast Food Culture:

•    Convenience and Accessibility: Fast food is often convenient and readily accessible, promoting its widespread consumption. These foods are typically high in calories and low in nutritional content.

• Large Portion Sizes: Fast-food establishments often offer larger portion sizes, contributing to excessive calorie intake in a single meal.

3. Sugar-Sweetened Beverages:

• Empty Calories: Beverages high in added sugars, such as sodas and sweetened juices, contribute to excess calorie consumption without providing essential nutrients.

• Liquid Calories: Consuming calories in liquid form may not induce the same feeling of fullness as solid foods, leading to additional calorie intake.

4. Snacking on Unhealthy Options:

- Mindless Snacking: Snacking on high-calorie, low-nutrient foods between meals can lead to overconsumption, especially when done mindlessly.

- Processed Snack Foods: Many commercially available snacks, such as chips and cookies, are energy-dense and lack nutritional value.

5. Lack of Whole Foods:

- Limited Fruits and Vegetables: Insufficient consumption of fruits and vegetables, which are nutrient-rich and lower in calories, contributes to an imbalance in the diet.

- Low-Fiber Intake: Diets lacking in whole foods often result in low fiber intake, affecting digestive health and satiety.

6. High-Fat and Fried Foods:

- Calorie-Dense Choices: Foods high in unhealthy fats and fried options are calorie-dense and can contribute to weight gain.

•	Inflammatory Effects: Diets rich in trans fats and saturated fats from fried foods may have inflammatory effects, impacting overall health.

7.	Cultural and Social Influences:

•	Social Norms: Cultural norms and societal trends may encourage the consumption of high-calorie, low-nutrient foods as part of social gatherings and celebrations.

•	Marketing Influence: Aggressive marketing of such foods can influence consumer choices and contribute to their widespread consumption.

8.	Limited Nutritional Education:

•	Lack of Awareness: Limited understanding of the nutritional content of foods may result in individuals making choices based on taste and convenience rather than considering their health impact.

•      Nutritional Literacy: Improving nutritional education and literacy empowers individuals to make informed choices and prioritize nutrient-dense options.

a) Addressing the consumption of high-calorie, low-nutrient foods involves promoting nutritional education, raising awareness about healthier alternatives, and fostering a shift toward whole, nutrient-dense foods. Encouraging individuals to make mindful and informed choices is essential for preventing obesity and promoting overall well-being.

## 2. Overeating and portion sizes

Overeating and the issue of portion sizes play a crucial role in the development and persistence of obesity.

These behavioral patterns involve consuming more calories than the body requires, leading to an energy imbalance and subsequent weight gain. Understanding the factors contributing to overeating and the role of portion sizes is essential for promoting healthier eating habits and weight management. Several factors contribute to these behaviors:

1.	Environmental Cues:

•	Large Portions: The prevalence of large portion sizes in restaurants, fast-food establishments, and packaged foods can lead individuals to consume more calories than needed.

•	Visual Cues: Visual cues, such as larger plates and oversized servings, may prompt individuals to eat more without being fully aware of the increased calorie intake.

2.	Emotional Eating:

•       Stress and Emotions: Emotional triggers, such as stress, boredom, or sadness, can lead to overeating as a way to cope with emotional discomfort.

•       Mindless Eating: Consuming food without paying attention to hunger and fullness cues, often associated with emotional eating, can lead to excessive calorie intake.

3.    Social Influences:

•       Social Gatherings: Social situations, celebrations, and gatherings often involve abundant food offerings, encouraging overeating in a communal setting.

•       Peer Pressure: Social pressure to conform to eating norms or finish large portions can contribute to overeating.

4.    Highly Palatable Foods:

•       Processed and Hyper-Palatable Foods: Highly processed and hyper-palatable foods, designed for maximum taste appeal, may lead individuals to consume larger quantities due to their addictive nature.

•	Craving and Reward System: The combination of sugar, fat, and salt in these foods can trigger cravings and disrupt the body's natural satiety signals.

5.	Lack of Mindful Eating:

•	Eating Speed: Rapid eating and not savoring food can lead to overeating, as the body may not have enough time to register fullness.

•	Distractions during Meals: Engaging in distractions such as watching TV or using electronic devices during meals can lead to mindless eating and overconsumption.

6.	Environmental Cues:

•	Food Advertising: Promotional activities and advertising, especially for energy-dense foods, can influence individuals to consume more than necessary.

• Food Accessibility: Easy access to snacks and convenience foods may contribute to impulsive eating and larger portion sizes.

7. Lack of Hunger Awareness:

• Eating Despite Fullness: Disregarding signals of fullness and continuing to eat may result from various factors, including cultural expectations to finish meals.

• Psychological Hunger: Distinguishing between physical hunger and psychological cues is essential to prevent unnecessary overeating.

8. Meal Frequency and Snacking:

• Frequent Snacking: Regular snacking, especially on high-calorie snacks, can contribute to an increased overall daily calorie intake.

•	Large Snack Portions: Consuming large portions during snack times may add substantial calories to the diet.

9.	Portion Distortion:

•	Perception of Normal Portion Sizes: Distorted perceptions of what constitutes a normal portion size can contribute to overeating.

•	Restaurant Portion Sizes: Oversized portions served at restaurants may contribute to the normalization of larger serving sizes.

Addressing overeating and portion sizes involves adopting mindful eating practices, promoting awareness of hunger and fullness cues, and creating environments that support healthier eating habits. Educating individuals about appropriate portion sizes, encouraging mindful eating, and fostering a positive relationship with food are crucial steps in preventing and managing obesity.

## ❖ Physical activity

Physical activity, or the lack thereof, is a fundamental aspect influencing weight management and overall well-being. Adequate physical activity is essential for maintaining a healthy body weight, improving cardiovascular health, and preventing various chronic conditions. Understanding the role of physical activity, its benefits, and the barriers to engagement is crucial for promoting a more active lifestyle.

1.    Benefits of Regular Physical Activity:

•    Calorie Expenditure: Engaging in physical activity helps burn calories, contributing to a healthy energy balance and weight management.

•	Cardiovascular Health: Regular exercise improves cardiovascular health by strengthening the heart, enhancing circulation, and lowering the risk of heart diseases.

•	Metabolic Health: Physical activity plays a key role in regulating blood sugar levels and improving insulin sensitivity, reducing the risk of type 2 diabetes.

•	Mental Well-being: Exercise is linked to improved mood, reduced stress, and enhanced cognitive function, promoting mental well-being.

•	Muscle and Bone Health: Weight-bearing activities contribute to the maintenance of strong muscles and bones, reducing the risk of osteoporosis and frailty.

2.	Sedentary Lifestyle and Health Risks:

•	Consequences of Inactivity: Prolonged periods of sitting and a sedentary lifestyle are associated with increased health risks, including obesity, cardiovascular diseases, and musculoskeletal issues.

•	Impact on Metabolism: Lack of physical activity can contribute to a slower metabolism, making it more challenging to maintain a healthy weight.

3.	Barriers to Physical Activity:

•	Time Constraints: Busy schedules and time constraints are common barriers to regular physical activity. Individuals may struggle to find time for exercise amidst other priorities.

•	Lack of Motivation: A lack of motivation or interest in physical activities can hinder individuals from incorporating regular exercise into their routines.

• Environmental Factors: Limited access to safe and convenient spaces for physical activity, such as parks or gyms, can be a barrier, particularly in certain communities.

• Health Conditions: Physical limitations or certain health conditions may restrict the ability to engage in certain types of exercise, making it challenging for some individuals.

• Perceived Difficulty: The perception that exercise is difficult or requires a high level of fitness can discourage individuals, especially beginners, from starting a regular exercise routine.

4.    Types of Physical Activity:

• Cardiovascular Exercise: Activities such as walking, running, cycling, and swimming contribute to cardiovascular fitness and calorie expenditure.

•       Strength Training: Incorporating resistance training with weights or bodyweight exercises helps build and maintain muscle mass, supporting overall health.

•       Flexibility and Balance: Practices like yoga or stretching exercises enhance flexibility, balance, and joint mobility.

5.      Incorporating Physical Activity into Daily Life:

•       Active Commuting: Choosing active modes of transportation, such as walking or cycling, integrates physical activity into daily routines.

•       Short, Regular Sessions: Breaking down exercise into shorter, more frequent sessions can be as beneficial as longer workouts, making it more manageable for individuals with busy schedules.

• Family and Social Activities: Engaging in physical activities with family or friends can make exercise more enjoyable and increase adherence.

6. Physical Activity Guidelines:

• Global Recommendations: Following global physical activity guidelines, such as those provided by health organizations, helps individuals understand the recommended duration and intensity of exercise for optimal health.

• Adaptation to Abilities: Tailoring physical activity to individual fitness levels and preferences increases the likelihood of adherence.

7. Educational and Support Programs:

• Workplace Wellness Programs: Employers can promote physical activity through workplace wellness initiatives, including fitness classes, ergonomic adjustments, and encouragement of active breaks.

• Community Programs: Local communities can organize fitness classes, sports leagues, and recreational activities to encourage residents to be physically active.

Promoting physical activity involves addressing barriers, providing education on the benefits, and creating environments that support active living. Encouraging individuals to find activities they enjoy and making physical activity an integral part of daily life are key strategies in preventing obesity and promoting overall health.

### 1. Sedentary Lifestyle and Its Consequences:

A sedentary lifestyle, characterized by prolonged periods of sitting and low levels of physical activity, has profound implications for overall health and well-being. The consequences of a sedentary lifestyle extend beyond the immediate physical effects, impacting various aspects of health and contributing to the development of chronic conditions. Understanding these consequences is crucial for promoting awareness and encouraging individuals to adopt more active lifestyles.

1. Obesity and Weight Gain:

• Energy Imbalance: Prolonged sitting reduces the number of calories burned, leading to an energy imbalance when combined with excessive calorie intake. This imbalance contributes to weight gain and obesity.

•    Metabolic Effects: Sedentary behavior can lead to metabolic changes, including reduced insulin sensitivity and altered glucose metabolism, increasing the risk of type 2 diabetes.

2.    Cardiovascular Health:

•    Increased Risk of Cardiovascular Diseases: A sedentary lifestyle is a major risk factor for cardiovascular diseases. Lack of regular physical activity contributes to elevated blood pressure, cholesterol levels, and atherosclerosis.

•    Reduced Cardiovascular Fitness: Insufficient physical activity leads to reduced cardiovascular fitness, limiting the heart's ability to efficiently pump blood and oxygen to the body.

3.    Musculoskeletal Issues:

•    Muscle Atrophy and Weakness: Lack of movement can lead to muscle atrophy and weakness, affecting posture, stability, and overall musculoskeletal health.

•	Joint Stiffness and Pain: Sedentary behavior contributes to joint stiffness and increased susceptibility to musculoskeletal pain, particularly in the back, neck, and joints.

4.	Mental Health Impacts:

•	Increased Risk of Depression and Anxiety: Sedentary lifestyles are associated with an increased risk of mental health issues, including depression and anxiety.

•	Cognitive Decline: Insufficient physical activity is linked to cognitive decline and an increased risk of neurodegenerative conditions such as Alzheimer's disease.

5.	Reduced Immune Function:

•	Suppressed Immune Response: Sedentary behavior can suppress the immune system, making individuals more susceptible to infections and illnesses.

•	Inflammation: Chronic inflammation associated with a sedentary lifestyle contributes to various health problems, including autoimmune conditions.

6.	Increased Risk of Chronic Diseases:

•	Type 2 Diabetes: Sedentary behavior is a significant risk factor for the development of type 2 diabetes due to impaired glucose metabolism.

•	Certain Cancers: Studies suggest that prolonged sitting is associated with an increased risk of certain cancers, including colorectal, breast, and ovarian cancers.

7.	Poor Posture and Back Issues:

•      Spinal Misalignment: Extended periods of sitting can lead to poor posture and spinal misalignment, contributing to back pain and discomfort.

•      Disk Compression: Sedentary behavior may increase the risk of intervertebral disk compression and herniation.

8.    Sleep Disturbances:

•      Insomnia and Poor Sleep Quality: Sedentary lifestyles are linked to disrupted sleep patterns, leading to difficulties falling asleep and poor sleep quality.

•      Daytime Sleepiness: Lack of physical activity can contribute to daytime sleepiness and fatigue.

9.    Social and Emotional Impact:

•      Isolation and Reduced Social Interaction: Sedentary behaviors, often associated with screen time, may contribute to social isolation and reduced face-to-face interactions.

•	Impact on Emotional Well-being: Physical inactivity can negatively affect emotional well-being, contributing to stress and decreased overall life satisfaction.

10.	Shortened Lifespan:

•	Increased Mortality Risk: Studies consistently show that a sedentary lifestyle is associated with an increased risk of premature death. Lack of physical activity is a significant contributor to reduced life expectancy.

Promoting awareness of the consequences of a sedentary lifestyle is crucial for encouraging individuals to incorporate more movement into their daily routines. Adopting regular physical activity and reducing prolonged sitting are essential steps in mitigating these health risks and improving overall well-being.

## 2. Lack of Regular Exercise:

The absence of regular exercise, characterized by insufficient physical activity, has far-reaching consequences on both physical and mental health. Regular exercise is essential for maintaining overall well-being, and the lack of it can lead to various health issues. Understanding the impacts of insufficient physical activity is crucial for motivating individuals to incorporate regular exercise into their lifestyles.

1.    Weight Management and Obesity:

•    Calorie Imbalance: Lack of regular exercise contributes to an imbalance between calories consumed and calories expended, leading to weight gain and an increased risk of obesity.

•    Reduced Metabolic Rate: Inactivity can lead to a decrease in metabolic rate, making it more challenging to maintain a healthy weight.

2.    Cardiovascular Health:

•    Increased Risk of Heart Diseases: Insufficient physical activity is a significant risk factor for cardiovascular diseases, including coronary artery disease, heart attacks, and strokes.

•    Elevated Blood Pressure and Cholesterol Levels: Lack of regular exercise contributes to elevated blood pressure and cholesterol levels, further impacting cardiovascular health.

3.    Type 2 Diabetes:

•    Insulin Resistance: Inactivity contributes to insulin resistance, a key factor in the development of type 2 diabetes.

•    Impaired Glucose Metabolism: Regular exercise improves glucose metabolism, reducing the risk of developing diabetes.

4.    Muscle Atrophy and Weakness:

•    Loss of Muscle Mass: Lack of exercise leads to muscle atrophy and weakness, impacting overall strength, endurance, and functional capacity.

•    Reduced Joint Stability: Weak muscles can contribute to joint instability and an increased risk of injuries.

5.    Bone Health:

•    Reduced Bone Density: Inactivity is associated with decreased bone density, increasing the risk of osteoporosis and fractures.

•    Impaired Joint Health: Lack of weight-bearing exercise hinders joint health and may contribute to conditions like arthritis.

6.    Mental Health Impacts:

•	Increased Risk of Depression and Anxiety: Regular exercise is linked to improved mood and reduced risk of depression and anxiety.

•	Cognitive Function: Physical activity enhances cognitive function, and lack of exercise may contribute to cognitive decline and impaired mental acuity.

7.	Poor Sleep Quality:

•	Insomnia and Sleep Disorders: Lack of physical activity is associated with sleep disturbances, including insomnia and poor sleep quality.

•	Disrupted Sleep Patterns: Regular exercise helps regulate sleep patterns and promotes better overall sleep.

8.	Increased Risk of Chronic Diseases:

•      Certain Cancers: Inactivity is a risk factor for certain cancers, including breast, colon, and prostate cancers.

•      Chronic Respiratory Conditions: Lack of exercise is associated with an increased risk of chronic respiratory conditions, such as chronic obstructive pulmonary disease (COPD).

9.     Metabolic Syndrome:

•      Cluster of Risk Factors: Sedentary behavior contributes to the development of metabolic syndrome, a cluster of risk factors including abdominal obesity, insulin resistance, and high blood pressure.

•      Systemic Health Implications: Metabolic syndrome increases the risk of heart diseases, stroke, and type 2 diabetes.

10.   Quality of Life and Longevity:

•	Decreased Quality of Life: Lack of regular exercise is linked to a decreased quality of life, affecting physical function, mental well-being, and overall life satisfaction.

•	Reduced Lifespan: Studies consistently show that insufficient physical activity is associated with a higher risk of premature mortality.

Encouraging regular exercise is paramount for mitigating these health risks and promoting overall well-being. Establishing enjoyable and sustainable exercise routines, incorporating both cardiovascular and strength-training activities, is essential for maintaining good health throughout life.

# CHAPTER 5: SOCIOECONOMIC FACTORS

Socioeconomic factors play a significant role in shaping individual behaviors, access to resources, and overall health outcomes, including the risk of obesity. Understanding the complex interplay between socioeconomic status and obesity is crucial for addressing disparities and implementing effective strategies to promote healthier lifestyles.

1.    Income and Education:

•    Access to Healthy Foods: Individuals with higher incomes often have better access to a variety of fresh and nutritious foods. Lower-income communities may face food deserts with limited access to affordable, healthy options.

•    Nutritional Knowledge: Higher education levels are often associated with better nutritional knowledge, influencing food choices and dietary habits.

2.    Food Insecurity:

•    Limited Access to Nutritious Foods: Economic challenges can lead to food insecurity, where individuals may prioritize more affordable, calorie-dense but nutrient-poor options, contributing to obesity.

•    Stress and Coping Mechanisms: Food insecurity, often associated with economic hardship, can lead to stress-induced overeating and reliance on energy-dense foods.

3.    Built Environment:

•    Neighborhood Infrastructure: Socioeconomic status can influence the built environment, with lower-income neighborhoods often lacking safe spaces for physical activity, such as parks and recreational facilities.

•      Walkability and Accessibility: Limited walkability and accessibility to exercise opportunities may contribute to sedentary lifestyles in economically disadvantaged areas.

4.    Occupational Factors:

•      Job Type and Work Conditions: Certain occupations, particularly those with low wages and long hours, may limit opportunities for physical activity. Sedentary jobs contribute to a more inactive lifestyle.

•      Workplace Wellness Programs: Higher-income individuals may have access to workplace wellness programs, promoting physical activity and healthier lifestyles.

5.    Advertising and Marketing:

•	Targeted Marketing: Lower-income populations are often targets of aggressive marketing for low-cost, high-calorie, and processed foods, influencing dietary choices.

•	Media Influence: Socioeconomic factors can affect media literacy, influencing individuals' ability to critically evaluate food marketing messages.

6.	Cultural and Social Norms:

•	Cultural Perceptions of Body Image: Socioeconomic factors can influence cultural perceptions of body image, impacting attitudes towards weight and contributing to body weight norms.

•	Social Influences: Economic status may shape social norms related to physical activity and dietary patterns within communities.

7.	Access to Healthcare:

• Preventive Healthcare Services: Higher-income individuals often have better access to preventive healthcare services, including nutrition counseling and weight management support.

• Treatment and Intervention: Socioeconomic disparities can affect the availability and utilization of obesity treatment options, leading to unequal health outcomes.

8. Education and Health Literacy:

• Understanding Health Information: Higher educational attainment is often associated with better health literacy, influencing an individual's ability to understand and apply health-related information.

• Engagement in Health-promoting Behaviors: Education can empower individuals to engage in health-promoting behaviors, including regular exercise and balanced nutrition.

9.    Stress and Mental Health:

•    Psychosocial Stressors: Socioeconomic challenges, such as financial strain and employment instability, contribute to psychosocial stressors linked to obesity.

•    Mental Health Access: Disparities in mental health resources and access to mental health services may impact coping mechanisms, including emotional eating.

10.   Government Policies and Initiatives:

•    Public Health Interventions: Government policies and public health initiatives can address socioeconomic factors by implementing programs that promote healthy behaviors, improve food access, and create supportive environments.

- Social Safety Nets: Robust social safety nets may alleviate economic stressors, indirectly influencing obesity rates by reducing stress-related behaviors.

Addressing socioeconomic factors in the context of obesity requires a comprehensive approach that considers structural inequalities, promotes economic well-being, and implements policies fostering equitable access to resources and opportunities for health. Strategies should focus on creating environments that support healthy living, regardless of socioeconomic status, to reduce obesity disparities.

## ❖ Economic Disparities and Their Impact on Diet:

Economic disparities significantly influence dietary patterns, creating unequal access to nutritious foods and contributing to disparities in obesity rates. The availability of resources, purchasing power, and educational opportunities influence the quality of diets individuals can afford and, consequently, their overall health. Understanding the impact of economic disparities on diet is crucial for addressing health inequalities and promoting healthier food choices.

1.    Food Affordability and Availability:

•    Limited Access to Fresh Produce: Lower-income individuals may face challenges accessing fresh fruits, vegetables, and other nutrient-dense foods due to financial constraints and a lack of nearby grocery stores.

•    Reliance on Processed Foods: Economic constraints may lead to a higher reliance on processed and energy-dense foods, which are often more affordable but less nutritious.

## 2.    Food Deserts:

•    Geographic Disparities: Lower-income neighborhoods may lack access to supermarkets and grocery stores, creating food deserts where residents have limited options for purchasing healthy foods.

•    Convenience Store Options: In food deserts, convenience stores may be the primary source of groceries, offering a limited selection of nutritious foods.

## 3.    Nutritional Knowledge and Education:

•    Educational Disparities: Economic disparities often correlate with differences in educational attainment. Limited education can result in lower nutritional literacy, impacting the ability to make informed and healthy food choices.

•      Influence on Dietary Habits: Higher educational levels are associated with healthier dietary habits, as individuals with more education may be more aware of the importance of balanced nutrition.

4.    Price Disparities in Healthy Foods:

•      Cost of Fresh Produce: The perceived high cost of fresh produce and healthier food options may discourage lower-income individuals from incorporating these items into their diets.

•      Affordability of Processed Foods: Processed and calorie-dense foods are often more affordable, leading to a higher consumption of energy-dense, nutrient-poor options.

5.    Cultural and Social Influences:

•      Cultural Food Preferences: Cultural factors may influence dietary preferences, and traditional, healthier foods may be perceived as less accessible or affordable.

•      Social Norms and Peer Influence: Economic disparities can shape social norms related to food choices, and individuals may be influenced by peers or communities where unhealthy food options are more prevalent.

6.    Fast Food Consumption:

•      Convenience and Affordability: Fast food, often high in calories and low in nutritional value, may be more accessible and affordable for those with limited financial resources.

•      Impact on Dietary Quality: Frequent consumption of fast food can contribute to poor dietary quality and increased risk of obesity.

7.    Marketing and Advertising:

•	Targeting Lower-Income Consumers: Advertising of inexpensive, energy-dense foods is often targeted towards lower-income populations, influencing food choices and contributing to less healthy diets.

•	Limited Exposure to Healthier Options: Lower-income individuals may have limited exposure to marketing promoting healthier food choices.

8.	Access to Cooking Facilities:

•	Limited Kitchen Resources: Economic constraints may result in limited access to cooking facilities or utensils, leading individuals to rely on convenient, processed, and less nutritious food options.

•	Impact on Meal Preparation: Limited resources may hinder the ability to prepare fresh and healthy meals at home, influencing dietary habits.

9.    Food Assistance Programs:

•    Accessibility and Nutritional Quality: Participation in food assistance programs, such as SNAP (Supplemental Nutrition Assistance Program), can influence the types of foods individuals can afford, with potential implications for dietary quality.

•    Addressing Gaps in Food Access: Strengthening food assistance programs to prioritize nutritional quality can help address disparities in food access.

10.  Community Resources and Support:

•    Community Initiatives: Economic disparities impact the availability of community resources, such as nutrition education programs, community gardens, and food cooperatives, which can enhance access to healthier foods.

- Collaborative Efforts: Collaborative efforts between communities, local governments, and businesses can work to reduce economic disparities and improve access to nutritious foods.

Addressing the impact of economic disparities on diet requires multifaceted approaches, including policy changes, community interventions, and educational initiatives. Efforts to increase access to affordable, nutritious foods and promote nutritional education can contribute to reducing diet-related health inequalities.

## ❖ Access to Health Care and Obesity Prevention:

Access to healthcare plays a pivotal role in obesity prevention, as it influences individuals' ability to receive timely and appropriate interventions, guidance, and support for maintaining a healthy weight.

Addressing healthcare disparities is essential for implementing effective obesity prevention strategies and promoting overall well-being.

1.    Preventive Services:

•    Regular Health Check-ups: Access to routine medical check-ups allows for the early detection of potential weight-related issues and facilitates preventive interventions.

•    Screening and Counseling: Healthcare providers can offer screening for obesity and provide counseling on nutrition, physical activity, and lifestyle modifications to prevent weight gain.

2.    Nutritional Guidance:

•    Dietary Counseling: Access to nutritionists or dietitians can help individuals receive personalized dietary guidance, fostering healthier eating habits and preventing obesity.

•	Education on Healthy Eating: Healthcare professionals can educate patients on the importance of a balanced diet and how to make informed food choices.

3.	Physical Activity Programs:

•	Exercise Prescription: Healthcare providers can prescribe exercise tailored to individual needs, considering factors like age, health status, and personal preferences.

•	Referral to Exercise Specialists: Access to exercise specialists or physical therapists can enhance the effectiveness of physical activity interventions.

4.	Behavioral Interventions:

•	Cognitive-Behavioral Therapy: Access to behavioral health services, including cognitive-behavioral therapy, can address emotional and psychological factors contributing to obesity, promoting healthier behaviors.

•	Behavioral Modification Programs: Healthcare professionals can recommend or provide access to programs focusing on behavior modification to support sustainable lifestyle changes.

5.	Medical Monitoring and Management:

•	Monitoring Health Metrics: Regular healthcare visits allow for the monitoring of weight, blood pressure, and other health metrics, facilitating early intervention and management.

•	Medication Management: In some cases, medications may be prescribed to manage obesity-related conditions. Regular medical oversight ensures appropriate use and monitoring of medication effects.

6.    Access to Bariatric Surgery:

•    Evaluation and Consultation: For individuals with severe obesity, access to bariatric surgery consultations allows for a comprehensive assessment of risks and benefits.

•    Multidisciplinary Approach: Bariatric surgery programs often involve a multidisciplinary team, including dietitians, psychologists, and surgeons, to support pre- and post-operative care.

7.    Health Education Programs:

•    Community-Based Education: Accessible health education programs within communities can provide information on obesity prevention, promoting awareness and empowering individuals to make healthier choices.

• School-Based Initiatives: Integrating health education into schools can contribute to the development of lifelong healthy habits, including proper nutrition and regular physical activity.

8. Cultural Competency and Sensitivity:

• Culturally Tailored Interventions: Healthcare providers should offer culturally sensitive interventions that consider the diverse needs and preferences of various populations.

• Language Accessibility: Ensuring language accessibility in healthcare settings enhances communication and understanding, facilitating effective obesity prevention strategies.

9. Telehealth Services:

• Remote Consultations: Telehealth services can increase access to healthcare professionals, especially for individuals in remote or underserved areas, providing guidance on obesity prevention.

•    Virtual Support Groups: Telehealth platforms can facilitate virtual support groups, connecting individuals with similar goals and challenges for mutual encouragement.

10.   Collaboration with Community Resources:

•    Partnerships with Community Organizations: Healthcare providers can collaborate with community organizations to enhance access to resources, such as healthy food options, recreational facilities, and wellness programs.

•    Integration with Local Initiatives: Integrating healthcare efforts with existing local initiatives and community-driven programs strengthens obesity prevention strategies.

Improving access to healthcare services is integral to a comprehensive approach to obesity prevention. By addressing healthcare disparities, promoting preventive services, and fostering community collaborations, it is possible to create a supportive environment for individuals to achieve and maintain a healthy weight.

❖ **Education and Awareness Regarding Healthy Lifestyle Choices:**

Education and awareness initiatives are fundamental components of obesity prevention, empowering individuals to make informed decisions about their lifestyles. By promoting understanding of healthy choices, nutritional literacy, and the importance of physical activity, these efforts contribute to building a foundation for long-term well-being.

1.    School-Based Programs:

•    Nutrition Education: Integrating nutrition education into school curricula helps students develop a foundational understanding of healthy eating habits and the impact on overall health.

•    Physical Education: Robust physical education programs encourage regular physical activity and teach essential skills for maintaining an active lifestyle.

2.    Community Workshops and Seminars:

•    Health Literacy Workshops: Conducting workshops on health literacy equips community members with knowledge about nutrition, the importance of balanced diets, and the risks of obesity.

•	Interactive Seminars: Engaging seminars on healthy living, facilitated by healthcare professionals, nutritionists, and fitness experts, can inspire behavior change.

3.	Media Campaigns:

•	Public Service Announcements (PSAs): Media campaigns, including PSAs, can disseminate information about the benefits of healthy eating and physical activity to a broad audience.

•	Social Media Platforms: Utilizing social media platforms for health promotion campaigns reaches diverse demographics and encourages the sharing of health-related information.

4.	Online Resources and Apps:

•	Educational Websites: Accessible online resources provide information on nutrition, exercise, and obesity prevention, allowing individuals to educate themselves at their own pace.

• Health Apps: Mobile applications that offer guidance on healthy eating, exercise routines, and lifestyle choices provide practical tools for individuals seeking to adopt healthier habits.

5. Workplace Wellness Programs:

• Health Screenings: Incorporating health screenings as part of workplace wellness programs raises awareness of individual health metrics and encourages proactive health management.

• Educational Lunch-and-Learn Sessions: Organizing educational sessions during work hours informs employees about healthy lifestyle choices, fostering a culture of well-being.

6. Community Engagement Events:

• Health Fairs: Community health fairs provide a platform for local healthcare providers, nutritionists, and fitness experts to offer information, screenings, and demonstrations.

• Fitness Challenges: Organizing community-wide fitness challenges encourages participation and promotes a sense of collective responsibility for health.

7. Printed Materials:

• Pamphlets and Brochures: Distributing informative materials in clinics, community centers, and schools offers tangible resources for individuals to learn about healthy lifestyle choices.

• Posters and Infographics: Visual aids, such as posters and infographics, convey key messages about nutrition and physical activity in an easily digestible format.

8.     Partnerships with Educational Institutions:

•     Collaboration with Schools and Universities: Partnering with educational institutions allows for the integration of health education into academic curricula, reaching students across various age groups.

•     Internship Programs: Involving students in internship programs focused on health promotion fosters a culture of awareness and responsibility.

9.     Cultural Sensitivity in Education:

•     Tailored Messaging: Designing educational materials and campaigns that consider cultural diversity ensures that the information is relatable and resonates with various communities.

•     Incorporating Cultural Practices: Integrating traditional practices and cultural norms into health education programs respects diversity and enhances engagement.

10.  Peer Education Programs:

•      Student-Led Initiatives: Empowering students to lead initiatives promoting healthy lifestyles fosters a peer-to-peer approach, creating a supportive environment within educational institutions.

•      Community Health Ambassadors: Training community members as health ambassadors enables them to disseminate information and advocate for healthy living in their neighborhoods.

Education and awareness initiatives should emphasize the interconnectedness of nutrition, physical activity, and overall well-being. By fostering a culture of understanding and encouraging individuals to make informed choices, these programs play a crucial role in preventing obesity and promoting healthier lifestyles.

# CHAPTER 6: PSYCHOLOGICAL FACTORS

Psychological factors play a significant role in the development and management of obesity. Understanding the complex interplay between mental health and weight regulation is crucial for implementing effective strategies that address the psychological aspects contributing to obesity.

1.    Emotional Eating:

•    Stress-Induced Eating: Psychological stress can lead to emotional eating, where individuals use food as a coping mechanism to deal with emotions, contributing to overconsumption of calories.

•    Mindful Eating Practices: Promoting mindfulness and emotional awareness can help individuals develop healthier coping mechanisms, reducing reliance on food for emotional comfort.

2.    Body Image and Self-Esteem:

•    Negative Body Image: Poor body image and low self-esteem can contribute to unhealthy eating habits and a sedentary lifestyle, impacting overall well-being.

•    Promoting Positive Body Image: Educational programs and counseling that focus on building positive body image and self-esteem can support healthier behaviors.

3.    Binge Eating Disorder:

•    Binge Eating Patterns: Individuals with binge eating disorder may consume large amounts of food in a short period, leading to feelings of guilt and shame.

•    Cognitive-Behavioral Therapy (CBT): CBT, a therapeutic approach, has shown effectiveness in addressing binge eating disorder by targeting dysfunctional thought patterns and behaviors.

4.    Depression and Anxiety:

•    Impact on Eating Habits: Depression and anxiety can influence appetite, leading to changes in eating habits that may contribute to weight gain.

•    Integrated Mental Health Support: Integrated care that addresses both mental health and obesity can improve outcomes, including collaborative efforts between mental health professionals and healthcare providers.

5.    Trauma and Childhood Adversity:

•    Impact on Coping Mechanisms: Individuals who have experienced trauma or childhood adversity may develop maladaptive coping mechanisms, such as overeating, as a way to cope with emotional distress.

• Trauma-Informed Care: Implementing trauma-informed approaches in healthcare settings can enhance sensitivity and support for individuals with a history of trauma.

6. Social Isolation:

• Relationship with Emotional Eating: Social isolation and loneliness are linked to emotional eating and unhealthy dietary choices, as individuals may turn to food for comfort.

• Promoting Social Connection: Encouraging social engagement and community support can mitigate the impact of social isolation on psychological well-being.

7. Eating Disorders:

• Anorexia Nervosa and Bulimia Nervosa: These eating disorders are associated with distorted body image, extreme dieting, and unhealthy weight control behaviors.

•	Multidisciplinary Treatment: Addressing eating disorders requires a multidisciplinary approach involving mental health professionals, nutritionists, and medical practitioners.

8.	Cognitive Factors:

•	Dysfunctional Thought Patterns: Negative thought patterns related to food, body image, and weight can contribute to unhealthy behaviors.

•	Cognitive Restructuring: Cognitive-behavioral interventions that focus on restructuring maladaptive thoughts can support behavior change and improve psychological well-being.

9.	Impulsivity and Self-Control:

•	Impact on Eating Behavior: Impulsivity and a lack of self-control can lead to impulsive food choices and overeating.

•	Skill-Building Strategies: Interventions that enhance self-control and impulse regulation skills can be beneficial in promoting healthier eating behaviors.

10.	Motivation and Goal Setting:

•	Intrinsic vs. Extrinsic Motivation: Understanding individual motivations for weight management is essential. Intrinsic motivation, driven by personal values, tends to be more sustainable than extrinsic motivation.

•	Setting Realistic Goals: Encouraging individuals to set realistic and achievable goals fosters a sense of accomplishment and supports long-term behavior change.

Addressing psychological factors in obesity prevention involves a comprehensive approach that integrates mental health support, counseling, and behavioral interventions. By recognizing the nuanced relationship between psychological well-being and weight management, interventions can be tailored to address the unique needs of individuals, promoting both mental health and overall health.

## ❖ Emotional Eating and Its Connection to Obesity:

Emotional eating is a complex behavior where individuals turn to food as a means of coping with and managing their emotions. The link between emotional eating and obesity is significant, as the reliance on food for emotional comfort can lead to overconsumption of calories and contribute to weight gain. Understanding the dynamics of emotional eating is crucial for developing strategies to address its impact on obesity.

1.    Stress-Induced Eating:

•    Mechanism of Coping: Emotional eating often emerges as a coping mechanism in response to stress. When individuals experience stress, the brain may trigger a desire for comfort foods, leading to overeating.

•    Impact on Caloric Intake: Stress-induced emotional eating tends to involve the consumption of high-calorie, often unhealthy foods, contributing to an excess of calories.

2.    Mind-Body Connection:

•    Role of Hormones: Stress activates the release of hormones like cortisol, influencing appetite and food preferences. Emotional eating can disrupt the body's natural hunger and satiety signals.

•      Brain Reward System: The consumption of palatable foods during emotional eating triggers the brain's reward system, creating a cycle where individuals associate eating with emotional relief.

3.      Comfort Foods and Emotional Cravings:

•      Choice of Foods: Emotional eaters often seek out "comfort foods" that are high in sugar, fat, and carbohydrates. These foods may provide temporary emotional relief but contribute to long-term health issues.

•      Cravings and Emotional States: Emotional cravings can be linked to specific emotions, such as craving sweets when feeling sad or indulging in fatty foods when experiencing stress.

4.      Psychological Impact on Eating Habits:

•	Association with Emotions: Emotional eating creates an association between certain emotions and the act of eating. This association can lead to habitual patterns of eating in response to emotional triggers.

•	Dysregulated Eating Patterns: Chronic emotional eating can contribute to dysregulated eating patterns, making it challenging for individuals to maintain a balanced and healthy diet.

5.	Negative Emotional States and Obesity Risk:

•	Escaping Negative Emotions: Emotional eaters may use food as a way to temporarily escape negative emotions or stressors. This coping mechanism can contribute to a cycle of overeating and weight gain.

•	Long-Term Impact: Consistent reliance on emotional eating to manage negative emotions increases the risk of obesity and obesity-related health issues over time.

6.    Interventions for Emotional Eating:

•    Cognitive-Behavioral Therapy (CBT): CBT is an evidence-based approach that addresses the underlying thoughts and behaviors associated with emotional eating, helping individuals develop healthier coping strategies.

•    Mindfulness Practices: Mindfulness techniques, such as mindful eating, encourage individuals to be more aware of their emotions and eating habits, fostering a healthier relationship with food.

7.    Identifying Emotional Triggers:

•    Self-Reflection: Encouraging individuals to identify and reflect on their emotional triggers for eating allows them to recognize patterns and develop alternative coping mechanisms.

•	Journaling and Self-Monitoring: Keeping a food and emotion journal can help individuals track their emotional eating episodes, providing insights into the underlying emotional triggers.

8.	Building Emotional Resilience:

•	Stress Management Techniques: Teaching stress management techniques, such as deep breathing, meditation, or exercise, helps individuals build emotional resilience without resorting to emotional eating.

•	Seeking Support: Encouraging individuals to seek support from friends, family, or mental health professionals provides alternative outlets for emotional expression.

9.	Nutritional Education and Awareness:

•	Understanding Nutritional Impact: Educating individuals about the nutritional impact of emotional eating helps them make informed choices about food and fosters a greater awareness of the consequences.

•     Balanced Nutrition: Promoting a balanced and varied diet contributes to overall well-being and can reduce the reliance on specific foods for emotional comfort.

10.   Prevention Through Holistic Approaches:

•     Holistic Well-being: Holistic approaches that address mental, emotional, and physical well-being contribute to preventing emotional eating and obesity.

•     Lifestyle Changes: Encouraging individuals to adopt healthier lifestyles, including regular physical activity, sufficient sleep, and positive social connections, supports overall well-being and reduces reliance on emotional eating.

Recognizing emotional eating as a multifaceted behavior and addressing its connection to obesity involves a combination of psychological interventions, nutritional education, and holistic approaches to well-being. By providing individuals with tools to manage emotions effectively, it is possible to break the cycle of emotional eating and mitigate its impact on weight gain.

### ❖ Stress and Its Influence on Eating Behaviors:

Stress is a common and pervasive aspect of modern life, and its impact on eating behaviors is a complex interplay that often contributes to unhealthy dietary choices and can lead to weight-related issues. Understanding the relationship between stress and eating behaviors is essential for developing effective strategies to promote healthier coping mechanisms and prevent the negative effects on overall well-being.

1.    Hormonal Response to Stress:

•      Cortisol Release: Stress triggers the release of cortisol, often referred to as the "stress hormone." Elevated cortisol levels can influence appetite, leading to increased cravings for energy-dense and palatable foods.

•      Ghrelin and Leptin: Stress may disrupt the balance of hunger-regulating hormones, increasing ghrelin (appetite-stimulating) and reducing leptin (appetite-suppressing), contributing to overeating.

2.    Emotional Eating as a Coping Mechanism:

•    Comfort-Seeking Behaviors: During times of stress, individuals may turn to food as a coping mechanism to seek comfort and alleviate negative emotions.

•    Temporary Emotional Relief: Consuming high-calorie foods can provide a temporary sense of emotional relief, leading to a cycle of emotional eating.

3.    Cravings for Palatable Foods:

•    Preference for Energy-Dense Foods: Stress often leads to cravings for foods that are rich in sugars, fats, and carbohydrates, as these foods activate the brain's reward system.

•    Impact on Food Choices: Individuals under stress may be more inclined to choose less nutritious, processed foods that provide quick energy.

4.    Mindless Eating during Stress:

•	Distracted Eating: Stress can contribute to mindless or distracted eating, where individuals consume food without being fully aware of their eating patterns or portion sizes.

•	Lack of Satiety Signals: Stress-induced mindless eating may override the body's natural satiety signals, leading to excessive calorie consumption.

5.	Impact on Food Preferences:

•	Changes in Taste Preferences: Chronic stress may alter taste preferences, making individuals more inclined to choose sweeter, saltier, or more palatable foods.

•	Preference for Highly Processed Foods: The desire for convenience during stressful times can lead to an increased intake of highly processed and calorie-dense foods.

6.    Stress-Related Weight Gain:

•    Accumulation of Abdominal Fat: Chronic stress is associated with the accumulation of abdominal fat, which poses a higher risk for obesity-related health issues.

•    Effect on Metabolism: Prolonged stress may contribute to metabolic changes, such as insulin resistance, that can impact weight regulation.

7.    Psychological Factors:

•    Emotional Dysregulation: Stress can contribute to emotional dysregulation, making it difficult for individuals to manage their emotions in a healthy way.

•    Increased Craving Intensity: Psychological stress may intensify cravings, making it challenging for individuals to resist the allure of unhealthy foods.

8.    Social and Environmental Factors:

•    Social Eating Patterns: Stress can influence social eating patterns, leading to shared indulgence in unhealthy foods with friends or family members.

•    Accessibility of Comfort Foods: The availability and accessibility of comfort foods during stress may contribute to increased consumption.

9.    Coping Strategies:

•    Healthy vs. Unhealthy Coping Mechanisms: Individuals under stress may resort to either healthy coping mechanisms such as exercise or unhealthy ones like overeating. Promoting healthier coping strategies is crucial.

•    Mindfulness and Stress Reduction: Incorporating mindfulness practices and stress reduction techniques can help individuals manage stress without resorting to unhealthy eating habits.

10.    Interventions for Stress Management:

•      Cognitive-Behavioral Therapy (CBT): CBT can be effective in addressing the psychological aspects of stress and promoting healthier coping mechanisms.

•      Physical Activity: Regular physical activity is a powerful stress-reduction strategy that also positively influences overall health and well-being.

•      Mindfulness and Relaxation Techniques: Incorporating mindfulness meditation, deep breathing exercises, and other relaxation techniques can mitigate the physiological and psychological impact of stress.

Understanding the influence of stress on eating behaviors involves recognizing the intricate connections between physiological responses, psychological factors, and environmental influences. Interventions that focus on stress management, mindfulness, and the development of healthier coping mechanisms play a pivotal role in preventing stress-induced unhealthy eating patterns and their subsequent impact on weight.

## ❖ Mental Health Issues Contributing to Weight Gain:

Mental health issues can significantly impact weight regulation, often leading to weight gain and contributing to the complex interplay between psychological well-being and physical health. Recognizing and addressing the connection between mental health and weight is essential for developing comprehensive strategies that support individuals in managing both aspects of their well-being.

1.    Depression:

•      Changes in Appetite: Depression can lead to changes in appetite, with some individuals experiencing increased food intake and weight gain, while others may have a decreased appetite and unintentional weight loss.

•      Emotional Eating: Emotional eating as a coping mechanism during depressive episodes can contribute to unhealthy eating patterns and weight gain.

2.    Anxiety Disorders:

•      Stress-Induced Eating: Individuals with anxiety disorders may engage in stress-induced eating, particularly of high-calorie comfort foods, as a way to cope with heightened stress and anxiety.

•	Impact on Hormones: Chronic anxiety can disrupt hormonal balance, influencing appetite-regulating hormones and potentially leading to weight gain.

3.	Binge Eating Disorder (BED):

•	Episodes of Overeating: BED is characterized by recurrent episodes of consuming large amounts of food, often rapidly and to the point of discomfort, contributing to excessive caloric intake.

•	Weight Fluctuations: BED is associated with weight fluctuations, and individuals may experience weight gain over time due to the regular occurrence of binge-eating episodes.

4.	Post-Traumatic Stress Disorder (PTSD):

•	Emotional Dysregulation: PTSD can lead to emotional dysregulation, prompting individuals to use food as a way to self-soothe and manage distressing emotions.

•      Altered Eating Habits: Trauma survivors may develop altered eating habits, including emotional eating or avoidance of certain foods, which can impact weight.

5.      Medication Side Effects:

•      Antidepressants and Mood Stabilizers: Some medications prescribed for mental health conditions, such as certain antidepressants and mood stabilizers, may have side effects that contribute to weight gain.

•      Changes in Metabolism: Medications can affect metabolism and appetite regulation, leading to increased food intake and potential weight-related issues.

6.      Hormonal Imbalances:

•    Cortisol and Ghrelin Levels: Mental health issues can disrupt hormonal balance, with elevated cortisol levels from chronic stress influencing appetite and increased levels of ghrelin (hunger hormone) promoting overeating.

•    Insulin Resistance: Conditions like depression and anxiety have been linked to insulin resistance, which may contribute to weight gain and difficulty in weight management.

7.    Emotional Factors in Eating Disorders:

•    Body Image Concerns: Mental health issues, particularly those related to body image, can contribute to the development of eating disorders such as anorexia nervosa or bulimia nervosa, affecting weight significantly.

•    Compulsive Behaviors: Obsessive-compulsive tendencies related to body image and weight can result in extreme dieting or excessive exercise, impacting overall health.

8.    Chronic Stress:

•      Impact on Adiposity: Prolonged exposure to chronic stress can lead to an increase in visceral adiposity, particularly around the abdomen, increasing the risk of obesity-related health issues.

•      Elevated Insulin Levels: Chronic stress may contribute to elevated insulin levels, promoting fat storage and potentially leading to weight gain.

9.    Sleep Disorders:

•      Disruption of Circadian Rhythms: Sleep disorders, such as insomnia or sleep apnea, can disrupt circadian rhythms and hormonal balance, affecting appetite regulation and contributing to weight gain.

•	Impact on Emotional Well-being: Poor sleep quality is associated with mood disturbances, potentially influencing emotional eating patterns.

10.	Social Isolation and Loneliness:

•	Emotional Eating as a Coping Mechanism: Individuals experiencing social isolation or loneliness may turn to food as a means of emotional comfort, leading to overeating and weight gain.

•	Reduced Physical Activity: Social isolation can contribute to a sedentary lifestyle, impacting energy expenditure and potentially contributing to weight-related issues.

Addressing mental health issues that contribute to weight gain involves a holistic approach that integrates mental health interventions, therapeutic support, nutritional counseling, and lifestyle modifications. Collaborative efforts between mental health professionals and healthcare providers are crucial to developing personalized strategies that consider both mental well-being and weight management.

# CHAPTER 7: MEDICAL CONDITIONS

Several medical conditions can contribute to weight gain, affecting metabolic processes, hormonal balance, and overall health. Understanding these conditions is crucial for accurate diagnosis, appropriate treatment, and the development of effective strategies to manage weight-related issues associated with these medical conditions.

1.    Hypothyroidism:

•	Reduced Thyroid Function: Hypothyroidism is characterized by an underactive thyroid gland, leading to a decrease in the production of thyroid hormones.

•	Metabolic Impact: Reduced thyroid function can result in a slower metabolism, making it more challenging for individuals to maintain or lose weight.

2.	Polycystic Ovary Syndrome (PCOS):

•	Hormonal Imbalance: PCOS is marked by hormonal imbalances, including elevated levels of androgens (male hormones) and insulin resistance.

•	Impact on Weight: Insulin resistance can contribute to weight gain, particularly in the abdominal area, making weight management more challenging for individuals with PCOS.

3.    Cushing's Syndrome:

•    Excess Cortisol Production: Cushing's syndrome involves the overproduction of cortisol, often due to adrenal gland abnormalities or prolonged use of corticosteroid medications.

•    Weight Redistribution: Excess cortisol can lead to fat accumulation, especially around the face, neck, and abdomen, resulting in noticeable weight gain.

4.    Insulin Resistance:

•    Impaired Glucose Regulation: Insulin resistance occurs when cells do not respond effectively to insulin, leading to elevated blood sugar levels.

•    Increased Fat Storage: Insulin resistance can promote fat storage, particularly in visceral adipose tissue, contributing to weight gain.

5.    Hormonal Birth Control:

•    Potential for Weight Changes: Some individuals may experience weight changes when using hormonal birth control methods, though the impact varies.

•    Individual Responses: Weight gain or loss may be attributed to water retention, increased appetite, or hormonal changes, and the effect can differ among individuals.

6.    Antidepressant Medications:

•    Potential for Weight Gain: Certain antidepressant medications, especially selective serotonin reuptake inhibitors (SSRIs) and tricyclic antidepressants, may be associated with weight gain.

•    Individual Variability: Responses to medications vary, and weight changes can be influenced by factors such as metabolism, genetics, and lifestyle.

7.    Beta-Blockers:

•    Potential for Weight Gain: Beta-blockers, commonly prescribed for conditions like hypertension, can be associated with weight gain.

•    Metabolic Impact: Changes in metabolism and energy expenditure may contribute to weight-related side effects.

8.    Menopause:

•    Hormonal Changes: Menopause involves a decline in estrogen levels, which can lead to changes in fat distribution and metabolism.

•    Increased Abdominal Fat: Women experiencing menopause may notice an increase in abdominal fat, influencing overall body weight.

9.    Prader-Willi Syndrome:

• Genetic Disorder: Prader-Willi syndrome is a genetic disorder characterized by insatiable hunger and a slowed metabolism.

• Compulsive Overeating: Individuals with this syndrome often struggle with compulsive overeating, leading to significant weight gain.

10. Genetic Factors:

• Genetic Predisposition: Genetic factors can contribute to an individual's susceptibility to weight gain or obesity.

• Metabolic Variances: Variances in genes related to metabolism, appetite regulation, and fat storage can influence weight management.

11. Certain Psychiatric Medications:

• Weight-Related Side Effects: Some medications prescribed for psychiatric conditions, such as certain antipsychotics and mood stabilizers, may have weight-related side effects.

•	Individual Response: The impact on weight can vary among individuals, and monitoring is essential for minimizing adverse effects.

12.	Sleep Apnea:

•	Disordered Breathing during Sleep: Sleep apnea disrupts normal breathing patterns during sleep, affecting oxygen levels and metabolism.

•	Metabolic Impact: Sleep apnea has been associated with metabolic dysfunction, potentially contributing to weight gain.

13.	Gastrointestinal Disorders:

•	Digestive Issues: Certain gastrointestinal disorders, such as irritable bowel syndrome (IBS) or inflammatory bowel disease (IBD), can affect nutrient absorption and lead to weight changes.

•       Malabsorption: Malabsorption issues may result in nutrient deficiencies and unintended weight loss or gain.

Understanding the role of medical conditions in weight management is crucial for healthcare professionals to provide targeted interventions and support. Addressing underlying health issues, personalized treatment plans, and a multidisciplinary approach can help individuals manage their weight more effectively in the context of specific medical conditions.

## ❖ Hormonal Imbalances Affecting Metabolism:

Hormonal imbalances can significantly influence metabolism, impacting the body's ability to regulate energy expenditure and leading to changes in weight. Understanding the role of hormones in metabolism is crucial for addressing weight-related concerns associated with hormonal disturbances.

1.    Thyroid Hormones:

•    Hypothyroidism: In hypothyroidism, the thyroid gland produces insufficient thyroid hormones (T3 and T4), leading to a slowdown in metabolism.

•    Impact on Weight: Reduced thyroid function can result in weight gain, fatigue, and difficulty in losing weight despite dietary efforts.

2.    Insulin:

•    Insulin Resistance: Insulin is a key hormone in regulating blood sugar levels. Insulin resistance occurs when cells become less responsive to insulin, leading to elevated blood sugar levels.

•    Promotion of Fat Storage: Insulin resistance is associated with increased fat storage, particularly visceral fat, contributing to weight gain and making weight management challenging.

3.    Cortisol:

•    Stress Hormone: Cortisol is released in response to stress, playing a role in the body's fight-or-flight response.

•    Impact on Appetite: Chronic stress can lead to elevated cortisol levels, influencing appetite and potentially contributing to overeating and weight gain, particularly in the abdominal area.

4.    Ghrelin:

•    Hunger Hormone: Ghrelin is known as the "hunger hormone" and stimulates appetite.

•    Metabolic Impact: Imbalances in ghrelin levels may contribute to increased hunger and a higher likelihood of overeating, impacting overall energy balance.

5.   Leptin:

•   Satiety Hormone: Leptin signals satiety to the brain, indicating when the body has had enough food.

•   Resistance and Weight Gain: Leptin resistance can occur, diminishing its effectiveness and potentially leading to increased food intake and weight gain.

6.   Estrogen and Progesterone:

•   Menstrual Cycle Changes: Fluctuations in estrogen and progesterone during the menstrual cycle can influence water retention and impact weight.

•   Menopause: A decline in estrogen during menopause is associated with changes in fat distribution and metabolism, contributing to weight gain, particularly in the abdominal area.

7.    Testosterone:

•    Muscle Mass Maintenance: Testosterone plays a role in maintaining muscle mass, which influences overall metabolism.

•    Hormonal Decline with Age: Reductions in testosterone levels, especially in aging males, can contribute to decreased muscle mass and potential weight gain.

8.    Catecholamines (Epinephrine and Norepinephrine):

•    Fight-or-Flight Response: Catecholamines are released during the body's stress response, promoting increased heart rate and energy mobilization.

•    Metabolic Activation: While acute stress can temporarily boost metabolism, chronic stress may lead to dysregulation, impacting overall energy balance.

9.    Adiponectin:

•    Insulin Sensitivity: Adiponectin influences insulin sensitivity and helps regulate glucose metabolism.

•    Metabolic Protection: Higher levels of adiponectin are associated with improved insulin sensitivity and a lower risk of metabolic issues.

10.  Triiodothyronine (T3):

•    Active Thyroid Hormone: T3 is the active form of thyroid hormone that plays a crucial role in regulating metabolism.

•    Caloric Expenditure: T3 influences the body's basal metabolic rate, impacting the number of calories burned at rest.

## 11.  Melatonin:

•     Sleep Regulation: Melatonin, known for its role in sleep regulation, can influence metabolic processes.

•     Impact on Weight Regulation: Disruptions in sleep patterns or inadequate sleep may affect melatonin levels, potentially impacting weight management.

## 12.  Peptide YY (PYY):

•     Satiety Signal: PYY is released in the digestive tract and signals satiety to the brain.

•     Appetite Regulation: Higher levels of PYY are associated with reduced appetite and may contribute to weight regulation.

Addressing hormonal imbalances affecting metabolism involves a comprehensive approach, including lifestyle modifications, dietary interventions, and, when necessary, medical interventions. Collaborating with healthcare professionals can help individuals navigate the complexities of hormonal influences on metabolism and develop personalized strategies for weight management.

### ❖ Medications with Potential Side Effects of Weight Gain:

Certain medications are associated with side effects that may include weight gain. It's important for individuals to be aware of these potential effects and discuss any concerns with their healthcare provider. Adjustments to medication or additional strategies may be considered to manage weight while ensuring the effectiveness of the prescribed treatment.

1.   Antidepressants:

•	Selective Serotonin Reuptake Inhibitors (SSRIs): Common SSRIs like fluoxetine, sertraline, and paroxetine may be linked to weight gain.

•	Tricyclic Antidepressants (TCAs): TCAs, including amitriptyline and nortriptyline, are associated with weight gain.

2.	Antipsychotics:

•	Olanzapine: Used to treat conditions like schizophrenia and bipolar disorder, olanzapine is known for its potential to cause significant weight gain.

•	Clozapine: Another antipsychotic, clozapine, is associated with weight gain and metabolic changes.

3.	Corticosteroids:

•	Prednisone: Corticosteroids like prednisone, used to treat various inflammatory conditions, may lead to fluid retention and increased appetite, potentially resulting in weight gain.

4.    Mood Stabilizers:

•    Lithium: Prescribed for mood disorders such as bipolar disorder, lithium is linked to weight gain and changes in metabolism.

•    Valproate: Another mood stabilizer, valproate, is associated with weight gain and metabolic effects.

5.    Antidiabetic Medications:

•    Insulin: While essential for managing diabetes, insulin therapy can be associated with weight gain, especially if blood sugar control improves.

•    Sulfonylureas: Some oral antidiabetic medications, like glyburide and glipizide, may cause weight gain.

6.    Beta-Blockers:

• Propranolol: Beta-blockers, used to treat conditions such as hypertension and migraines, can lead to modest weight gain.

7. Certain Antihistamines:

• Cyproheptadine: This antihistamine is sometimes prescribed to stimulate appetite and may contribute to weight gain.

8. Antiepileptic Drugs:

• Gabapentin: Used to treat seizures and nerve pain, gabapentin is associated with weight gain.

• Pregabalin: Another antiepileptic drug, pregabalin, may lead to increased appetite and weight gain.

9. Hormonal Contraceptives:

• Depot Medroxyprogesterone Acetate (DMPA): Injectable contraceptives like DMPA have been associated with weight gain in some individuals.

10.   Selective Estrogen Receptor Modulators (SERMs):

•      Tamoxifen: Used in breast cancer treatment, tamoxifen may cause weight gain as a side effect.

11.   Antidepressant/Mood Stabilizer Combinations:

•      Quetiapine: Sometimes used as an adjunct treatment in depression, quetiapine can contribute to weight gain.

12.   Antiretroviral Medications:

•      Protease Inhibitors: Some medications used in the treatment of HIV, such as certain protease inhibitors, may be associated with metabolic changes and weight gain.

13.   Antihypertensive Medications:

•      Calcium Channel Blockers: Medications like amlodipine, commonly prescribed for hypertension, may cause mild weight gain.

It's crucial for individuals taking these medications to communicate openly with their healthcare provider about any observed changes in weight or concerns about potential side effects. Healthcare providers can explore alternative medications, adjust dosages, or recommend lifestyle modifications to help manage weight while considering the overall therapeutic goals of the prescribed treatments. Regular monitoring and collaboration between patients and healthcare professionals are essential to achieving a balance between effective medication management and weight control.

❖ Impact of Certain Medical Conditions on Obesity Risk:

Several medical conditions can significantly impact an individual's risk of developing obesity. Understanding these associations is crucial for preventive measures, targeted interventions, and comprehensive healthcare management. Here are some medical conditions and their impact on obesity risk:

1.    Hypothyroidism:

•    Impact: Hypothyroidism, characterized by an underactive thyroid gland, can lead to a slower metabolism and weight gain.

•    Connection to Obesity: Reduced thyroid function may contribute to obesity, and individuals with hypothyroidism may find it challenging to maintain a healthy weight.

2.    Polycystic Ovary Syndrome (PCOS):

•      Impact: PCOS is associated with hormonal imbalances, insulin resistance, and difficulties in regulating blood sugar levels.

•      Connection to Obesity: Insulin resistance in PCOS can contribute to weight gain, particularly around the abdominal area, increasing the risk of obesity.

3.     Cushing's Syndrome:

•      Impact: Cushing's syndrome involves excess cortisol production, leading to metabolic disturbances.

•      Connection to Obesity: Elevated cortisol levels can promote fat accumulation, especially in the abdominal region, increasing the risk of obesity.

4.     Insulin Resistance:

•      Impact: Insulin resistance, a condition where cells become less responsive to insulin, can lead to elevated blood sugar levels.

•      Connection to Obesity: Insulin resistance is often associated with weight gain, as it promotes fat storage and contributes to the development of obesity.

5.    Prader-Willi Syndrome:

•      Impact: Prader-Willi syndrome is a genetic disorder characterized by insatiable hunger and a slow metabolism.

•      Connection to Obesity: Individuals with Prader-Willi syndrome often struggle with compulsive overeating, leading to obesity if not closely managed.

6.    Genetic Factors:

•      Impact: Genetic predisposition can influence an individual's susceptibility to obesity.

•	Connection to Obesity: Variations in genes related to metabolism, appetite regulation, and fat storage can contribute to an increased risk of obesity.

7.	Sleep Apnea:

•	Impact: Sleep apnea disrupts normal breathing during sleep, affecting oxygen levels and metabolism.

•	Connection to Obesity: Obesity is a common risk factor for sleep apnea, and the condition can exacerbate weight-related issues.

8.	Gastrointestinal Disorders:

•	Impact: Certain gastrointestinal disorders, such as irritable bowel syndrome (IBS) or inflammatory bowel disease (IBD), can affect nutrient absorption.

•	Connection to Obesity: Malabsorption issues may lead to

nutrient deficiencies, potentially influencing weight gain or loss.

9.    Genetic Syndromes:

•    Impact: Certain genetic syndromes, such as Down syndrome, may be associated with metabolic and hormonal differences.

•    Connection to Obesity: Individuals with certain genetic syndromes may be more prone to obesity due to these underlying factors.

10.   Psychiatric Disorders:

•    Impact: Conditions like depression and anxiety can influence eating habits and lifestyle.

•    Connection to Obesity: Emotional eating and changes in physical activity associated with psychiatric disorders may contribute to weight gain and obesity.

## 11.  Chronic Inflammation:

•    Impact: Chronic inflammation is associated with various medical conditions, including autoimmune disorders.

•    Connection to Obesity: Inflammation may disrupt metabolic processes and contribute to weight-related issues.

## 12.  Certain Hormonal Changes:

•    Impact: Hormonal changes during menopause or as a result of hormonal treatments can affect metabolism.

•    Connection to Obesity: Altered hormonal balance may contribute to weight gain, particularly in women experiencing menopause.

Recognizing the impact of these medical conditions on obesity risk allows for targeted interventions, personalized healthcare plans, and a holistic approach to both the underlying medical condition and weight management. It emphasizes the importance of collaborative care between healthcare providers to address the unique needs of individuals with these conditions and promote overall well-being.

# CHAPTER 8: CULTURAL AND SOCIAL INFLUENCES

Understanding the cultural and social factors that contribute to obesity is essential for developing effective strategies to address this complex health issue. Various aspects of culture and society play a significant role in shaping individuals' behaviors, attitudes, and access to resources related to nutrition and physical activity.

1.    Cultural Perceptions of Body Image:

•    Body Ideals: Cultural norms and ideals surrounding body image can influence individuals' perceptions of an ideal body shape, impacting their attitudes toward weight and appearance.

• Pressure and Stigma: Societal pressure to conform to certain body standards may contribute to body dissatisfaction and, in some cases, disordered eating behaviors.

2. Dietary Practices and Culinary Traditions:

• Food Choices: Cultural dietary practices and preferences can significantly impact individuals' food choices, influencing the types and amounts of food consumed.

• Traditional Foods: Diets rich in traditional, culturally significant foods may contribute to variations in nutritional patterns and caloric intake.

3. Social Norms and Eating Habits:

• Social Eating: Cultural norms often dictate social eating habits, influencing the frequency and types of meals shared with others.

• Portion Sizes: Cultural norms may play a role in determining acceptable portion sizes, affecting overall caloric intake.

4. Physical Activity Patterns:

• Cultural Activities: Cultural and social activities may influence the level of physical activity in a community, impacting energy expenditure.

• Work and Leisure Habits: Societal norms regarding work and leisure may influence how much time individuals dedicate to physical activity.

5. Economic Disparities:

• Access to Healthy Foods: Economic disparities can affect access to nutritious foods, with lower-income individuals facing challenges in affording fresh and healthy options.

• Food Deserts: Socioeconomic factors can contribute to the existence of food deserts—areas with limited access to grocery stores offering fresh produce.

6.    Food Marketing and Advertising:

•    Cultural Influences in Advertising: Cultural values and norms are often reflected in food marketing, influencing consumer preferences and choices.

•    Impact on Food Choices: Exposure to culturally tailored advertising may affect individuals' perceptions of certain foods and contribute to dietary habits.

7.    Family and Social Support:

•    Family Dynamics: Cultural values within families can influence dietary patterns, as meals and eating habits are often shared within a familial context.

•    Social Support: The level of social support for healthy lifestyle choices, including nutrition and physical activity, varies across cultures and communities.

8.   Educational Attainment:

•   Impact on Health Literacy: Educational disparities can affect health literacy, influencing individuals' understanding of nutrition and its impact on health.

•   Access to Information: Socioeconomic factors may influence access to educational resources related to healthy lifestyle choices.

9.   Cultural Celebrations and Festivals:

•   Traditional Events: Cultural celebrations often involve specific foods and culinary traditions, impacting dietary patterns during festive periods.

•   Impact on Caloric Intake: Festive occasions may lead to increased caloric intake due to the availability of special and often indulgent foods.

10.   Cultural Perspectives on Health:

•	Holistic Health Views: Cultural perspectives on health may encompass holistic well-being, considering factors beyond physical health, such as mental and spiritual aspects.

•	Impact on Lifestyle Choices: A holistic approach to health may influence lifestyle choices, including dietary patterns and engagement in physical activities.

11.	Gender Roles and Expectations:

•	Social Expectations: Cultural expectations related to gender roles may influence individuals' attitudes toward physical activity and body image.

•	Impact on Health Behaviors: Traditional gender norms may contribute to differences in health behaviors, including dietary choices and exercise habits.

## 12. Religious Practices and Dietary Restrictions:

•	Fasting and Dietary Observances: Religious practices, such as fasting, may impact individuals' dietary habits and nutrient intake.

•	Cultural Dietary Restrictions: Certain cultural and religious beliefs may dictate dietary restrictions, influencing food choices.

Understanding and addressing cultural and social influences on obesity requires a culturally competent and inclusive approach. Tailoring interventions to respect and incorporate diverse cultural perspectives is essential for promoting health equity and effectively addressing the multifaceted nature of obesity in various communities. Collaboration between healthcare providers, policymakers, and community leaders is crucial in developing culturally sensitive strategies for prevention and intervention.

## ❖ Cultural Norms and Attitudes Towards Body Image:

Cultural norms and attitudes towards body image vary significantly across societies, influencing individuals' perceptions of beauty, self-worth, and body acceptance. These cultural influences play a crucial role in shaping attitudes toward body image, impacting mental health, well-being, and behaviors related to diet and physical activity.

1.    Body Ideals and Beauty Standards:

•    Varied Cultural Standards: Different cultures uphold diverse ideals of beauty, with some emphasizing specific body shapes, sizes, or features.

•    Media Influence: Cultural beauty standards are often reinforced by media representations, influencing individuals' perceptions of an ideal body image.

2.    Cultural Perceptions of Thinness or Fullness:

•    Thin Ideal: Some cultures may prioritize a thin or slender body as the epitome of beauty, leading to societal pressures to conform to this ideal.

•    Cultural Appreciation of Full Figures: In contrast, other cultures may appreciate fuller figures, associating them with health, fertility, or cultural ideals of attractiveness.

3.    Cultural Traditions and Rituals:

•    Impact of Cultural Practices: Cultural traditions and rituals, such as ceremonies or dances, may celebrate specific body types or movements, influencing perceptions of beauty.

•    Cultural Symbols: Certain body types may be symbolically significant within cultural practices, impacting attitudes toward body image.

4.      Generational Shifts in Body Image Ideals:

•       Evolution of Beauty Ideals: Attitudes toward body image may evolve over generations, with younger generations potentially challenging or redefining traditional beauty standards.

•       Media and Globalization: Increased exposure to global media can contribute to shifts in cultural perceptions of beauty.

5.      Cultural Acceptance of Diverse Body Types:

•       Body Diversity Appreciation: Some cultures may have a more inclusive approach to body diversity, appreciating a range of shapes and sizes.

•       Inclusive Representation: Cultures that celebrate diversity may emphasize the importance of representation in media and advertising to reflect a broader spectrum of body types.

6.   Stigma and Discrimination:

•   Stigmatization of Certain Body Types: Cultural norms may contribute to the stigmatization of individuals with bodies that deviate from prevailing beauty ideals.

•   Impact on Mental Health: Stigma and discrimination based on body image can negatively impact mental health, contributing to conditions like body dysmorphic disorder or eating disorders.

7.   Gender and Body Image:

•   Cultural Expectations for Men and Women: Cultural norms often prescribe specific body ideals for men and women, reinforcing gender-specific expectations.

•	Changing Gender Norms: Societal shifts in gender norms may influence evolving perceptions of body image, challenging traditional expectations.

8.	Cultural Influences on Clothing and Fashion:

•	Fashion Industry Standards: Cultural influences on the fashion industry can impact the types of bodies that are portrayed as fashionable or desirable.

•	Clothing Sizes: Cultural variations in clothing sizes and fit can affect individuals' perceptions of their bodies and influence their body image.

9.	Social Media and Online Culture:

•	Globalization of Beauty Ideals: Social media platforms contribute to the globalization of beauty ideals, influencing cultural perceptions of attractiveness.

- Impact on Body Image: Exposure to curated images on social media may affect individuals' body satisfaction and contribute to unrealistic beauty standards.

10. Cultural Practices Related to Diet and Exercise:

- Traditional Diets: Cultural dietary practices may influence body weight and shape, contributing to variations in body image attitudes.

- Historical Perspectives: Cultural histories related to physical activity and exercise may shape contemporary attitudes toward body image and fitness.

11. Religious Beliefs and Body Image:

- Fasting and Religious Observances: Religious practices, such as fasting, may influence body weight and shape, impacting individuals' perceptions of their bodies.

•	Modesty and Body Covering: Cultural and religious beliefs regarding modesty and body covering may affect individuals' comfort with their own bodies.

12.	Cultural Approaches to Aging and Beauty:

•	Attitudes Toward Aging: Cultural perspectives on aging can influence attitudes toward body image, with some cultures valuing and celebrating aging bodies.

•	Cultural Beauty Rituals: Traditional beauty rituals tied to aging may impact perceptions of attractiveness and body image.

Navigating and addressing cultural norms and attitudes towards body image requires sensitivity, awareness, and an understanding of the diverse factors influencing individual experiences. Promoting body positivity, inclusivity, and fostering healthy conversations around body image can contribute to a more supportive cultural environment for individuals of all shapes, sizes, and backgrounds.

### ❖ Social Acceptance of Unhealthy Behaviors:

In various societies, certain unhealthy behaviors may become socially accepted or normalized, contributing to widespread health challenges. Understanding the factors that lead to the acceptance of these behaviors is crucial for developing interventions to promote healthier lifestyles. Here are some examples of socially accepted unhealthy behaviors:

1.    Sedentary Lifestyle:

•    Desk Jobs and Technology Use: Modern lifestyles often involve prolonged periods of sitting due to desk jobs and increased use of technology.

•	Social Acceptance: Sedentary behaviors may be socially accepted, with little emphasis on the importance of regular physical activity.

2.	Overconsumption of Processed Foods:

•	Convenience Foods: The availability and convenience of processed and fast foods contribute to their overconsumption.

•	Social Norms: Fast food consumption may be socially accepted, and the prevalence of unhealthy dietary patterns can normalize poor nutritional choices.

3.	Excessive Sugar and Sugary Drinks:

•	Sugar-Laden Diets: Diets high in added sugars contribute to various health issues, yet the consumption of sugary foods and beverages is often socially accepted.

•	Marketing Influence: Aggressive marketing of sugary products may contribute to their normalization.

4.	Tobacco and Smoking:

•	Social Smoking: Smoking, despite being a leading cause of preventable diseases, is still socially accepted in certain contexts.

•	Cultural Norms: Cultural and social factors may contribute to the acceptance of smoking, and efforts to discourage tobacco use face resistance.

5.	Excessive Alcohol Consumption:

•	Binge Drinking: Binge drinking and excessive alcohol consumption are prevalent in some social circles.

• Social Events: Alcohol is often a part of social events, and the normalization of heavy drinking can contribute to its social acceptance.

6. Lack of Sleep and Sleep Deprivation:

• Busy Lifestyles: A culture that values productivity may contribute to the acceptance of insufficient sleep.

• Workplace Expectations: Work demands and societal expectations may lead to the normalization of sacrificing sleep for other activities.

7. Unsafe Driving Practices:

• Distracted Driving: The use of mobile phones and other distractions while driving is socially accepted in some communities.

• Speeding and Reckless Driving: Certain risky driving behaviors may be tolerated or normalized, contributing to road safety issues.

8.    Stress and Burnout:

•    High-Stress Environments: In certain professions, high stress is accepted as part of the job, contributing to burnout.

•    Limited Work-Life Balance: Societal norms emphasizing constant productivity can lead to the acceptance of chronic stress.

9.    Inadequate Hydration:

•    Prevalence of Sugary Drinks: High consumption of sugary drinks may overshadow the importance of staying adequately hydrated with water.

•    Cultural Practices: Cultural practices that prioritize other beverages over water can contribute to inadequate hydration.

## 10.  Lack of Mental Health Awareness:

•	Stigma around Mental Health: Social stigma surrounding mental health concerns can prevent open discussions and hinder seeking help.

•	Normalization of Stress: Stress-related issues may be normalized, impacting mental health outcomes.

## 11.  Unhealthy Body Image Standards:

•	Pressure for Unrealistic Ideals: Societal norms and media portrayals often promote unrealistic body image ideals.

•	Acceptance of Extreme Measures: Extreme dieting or unhealthy weight control measures may be accepted in the pursuit of these ideals.

## 12.  Inattentiveness to Preventive Healthcare:

•	Limited Emphasis on Preventive Measures: A reactive approach to health may contribute to the acceptance of neglecting preventive healthcare measures.

•	Late Health Seeking Behaviors: Delayed health-seeking behaviors may be normalized, impacting early detection and intervention.

Addressing the social acceptance of unhealthy behaviors requires a comprehensive approach, involving education, policy changes, and community engagement. Promoting awareness, creating supportive environments, and challenging societal norms that contribute to the normalization of unhealthy behaviors are essential steps toward fostering healthier lifestyles.

## ❖ Peer Pressure and Its Role in Shaping Lifestyle Choices:

Peer pressure, the influence exerted by one's social peers, plays a significant role in shaping various aspects of an individual's life, including lifestyle choices. This influence can impact behaviors related to health, diet, physical activity, and other lifestyle factors. Understanding the dynamics of peer pressure is crucial for promoting positive choices and mitigating potential negative effects. Here's an exploration of peer pressure's role in shaping lifestyle choices:

1.    Dietary Choices:

•    Food Preferences: Peer groups can influence individuals' food preferences, leading to the adoption of certain dietary habits based on what is socially accepted.

- Eating Out and Fast Food: Peer pressure can contribute to frequenting fast-food establishments or making unhealthy food choices in social settings.

2. Physical Activity and Exercise:

- Group Exercise: The influence of peers may encourage or discourage participation in physical activities, sports, or exercise routines.

- Sedentary Lifestyle: Peer pressure can contribute to a sedentary lifestyle if the social group engages in activities that discourage physical movement.

3. Substance Use:

- Smoking and Alcohol Consumption: Peer pressure can be a powerful factor in the initiation and continuation of smoking or excessive alcohol consumption.

•	Drug Use: Influences from social circles may lead individuals to experiment with or engage in drug use.

4.	Body Image and Appearance:

•	Fashion and Appearance: Peer pressure can influence clothing choices and grooming habits, impacting body image perceptions.

•	Pressure for Conformity: Social pressure to conform to certain beauty standards may contribute to unhealthy weight control behaviors.

5.	Sleep Habits:

•	Socializing Late: Peer influence may lead individuals to adopt sleep patterns that align with their social circles, potentially sacrificing adequate sleep.

•	Work and Study Pressure: Academic or work-related pressures within peer groups may impact sleep duration and quality.

6.  Stress Management:

•  Coping Mechanisms: Peer pressure can shape the adoption of certain stress-coping mechanisms, either healthy or unhealthy, such as relying on substances or engaging in relaxation activities.

•  Work-Life Balance: Social norms within peer groups may influence how individuals manage and cope with stressors related to work or personal life.

7.  Social Media Influence:

•  Online Behavior: Peer pressure extends to online platforms, where individuals may be influenced by the lifestyle choices and behaviors of their peers on social media.

•	Body Image and Comparison: Social media can contribute to peer pressure related to body image, leading individuals to compare themselves to others.

8.	Academic and Career Choices:

•	Course Selection: Peer influence can impact the choice of academic courses or career paths based on what is perceived as socially desirable.

•	Professional Goals: Career aspirations may be influenced by the preferences and expectations of one's peer group.

9.	Risk-Taking Behavior:

•	Thrill-Seeking: Peer pressure can contribute to engaging in risky behaviors, such as extreme sports or adventurous activities, to fit in with a particular social group.

•	Resistance to Risk Aversion: Social circles that value risk-taking may exert pressure on individuals to resist risk-averse behaviors.

10.	Health and Wellness Habits:

•	Wellness Practices: Peer influence can extend to adopting wellness practices, such as mindfulness, meditation, or holistic health approaches.

•	Supportive Networks: Positive peer pressure within supportive networks may encourage healthy lifestyle choices and discourage unhealthy habits.

Understanding the dynamics of peer pressure involves acknowledging its potential positive and negative impacts. Encouraging positive peer influences, fostering open communication, and promoting a supportive social environment can contribute to healthier lifestyle choices among individuals influenced by their peers. Education and empowerment to make informed decisions in the face of peer pressure are essential components of promoting overall well-being.

# CHAPTER 9: CHILDHOOD AND EARLY-LIFE INFLUENCES

Early experiences during childhood significantly shape an individual's health, habits, and well-being. Various factors, including family environment, nutrition, education, and social interactions, play pivotal roles in laying the foundation for lifelong habits and health outcomes. Examining these childhood and early-life influences provides insights into promoting positive development and preventing potential challenges:

1.    Early Nutrition and Feeding Habits:

•    Breastfeeding vs. Formula Feeding: The choice between breastfeeding and formula feeding can influence early nutrition and impact a child's immune system and overall health.

•    Introduction to Solid Foods: Early exposure to a variety of nutritious solid foods contributes to the development of healthy eating habits.

2.    Family Environment:

•    Parental Modeling: Parents serve as role models, influencing a child's attitudes toward diet, physical activity, and overall lifestyle choices.

•    Family Dynamics: The family environment, including communication patterns and support systems, shapes a child's emotional and mental well-being.

3.    Educational Experiences:

•	Early Learning Environments: Quality early childhood education fosters cognitive and social development, laying the groundwork for future academic success.

•	Literacy and Numeracy: Exposure to literacy and numeracy in early childhood influences cognitive skills and can impact long-term academic achievements.

4.	Socialization and Peer Interactions:

•	Social Skills Development: Early interactions with peers contribute to the development of social skills, communication abilities, and the understanding of relationships.

•	Peer Influences: Positive or negative peer interactions during childhood can shape behaviors, preferences, and attitudes toward various activities.

5.    Physical Activity Patterns:

•    Active Play: Encouraging active play and physical activities in childhood establishes a foundation for a healthy lifestyle and can prevent sedentary habits.

•    Outdoor Exploration: Exposure to outdoor environments enhances physical and sensory development and promotes a connection with nature.

6.    Screen Time and Media Exposure:

•    Digital Media Habits: Early exposure to digital media and screen time can impact cognitive development, sleep patterns, and attention spans.

•    Educational Content: Thoughtful use of educational media can support learning and early cognitive development.

7.    Sleep Hygiene:

•      Establishing Sleep Routines: Early bedtime routines and consistent sleep patterns contribute to the development of healthy sleep hygiene.

•      Impact on Cognitive Function: Quality sleep during childhood is crucial for cognitive functioning, memory consolidation, and emotional regulation.

8.     Emotional Well-being:

•      Secure Attachments: Nurturing secure attachments during early childhood promotes emotional well-being and resilience.

•      Emotional Regulation Skills: Learning emotional regulation skills in childhood contributes to better mental health outcomes in later life.

9.     Family Nutrition and Mealtime Habits:

•      Family Meals: Regular family meals foster positive relationships, communication, and the development of healthy eating habits.

• Exposure to Nutrient-Rich Foods: Early exposure to a variety of nutrient-rich foods influences taste preferences and dietary choices.

10. Cultural and Ethnic Influences:

• Cultural Identity: Early exposure to cultural practices, traditions, and languages shapes a child's sense of identity and belonging.

• Cultural Diets: Traditional diets influenced by cultural norms contribute to nutritional habits during childhood.

11. Immunization and Preventive Healthcare:

• Vaccination Practices: Timely immunizations during childhood protect against infectious diseases and contribute to public health.

•      Regular Health Checkups: Early and regular healthcare checkups establish a foundation for preventive care and health monitoring.

12.   Parental Involvement and Support:

•      Encouragement and Guidance: Supportive parenting styles that encourage exploration, autonomy, and positive behaviors contribute to a child's overall development.

•      Emotional Support: Providing emotional support and a secure attachment fosters a sense of security and resilience in children.

Understanding the multifaceted influences during childhood and early life allows for targeted interventions to promote positive development, prevent health disparities, and support overall well-being throughout the lifespan. Early investments in health and education create a foundation for a healthier and more resilient future generation.

## ❖ Impact of Early Feeding Practices on Obesity Risk:

Early feeding practices play a crucial role in shaping a child's nutrition, metabolism, and overall health. These practices not only influence immediate growth and development but also have long-term implications for obesity risk. Examining the impact of early feeding practices provides insights into preventive strategies and interventions to promote healthy weight in childhood and beyond:

1.   Breastfeeding vs. Formula Feeding:

•    Breastfeeding Advantages: Breastfeeding provides numerous health benefits, including optimal nutrition, immune system support, and appropriate energy intake.

•      Reduced Obesity Risk: Studies suggest that breastfeeding is associated with a reduced risk of childhood obesity, potentially due to the regulation of infant appetite and the promotion of healthy weight gain.

2.     Introduction of Solid Foods:

•      Timely Introduction: The timing of introducing solid foods is crucial. Early introduction before 4-6 months may be associated with an increased risk of obesity.

•      Nutrient-Rich Choices: Offering nutrient-dense foods during the introduction of solids contributes to healthy growth and helps establish positive eating habits.

3.     Parental Feeding Practices:

•      Responsive Feeding: Parents who respond to hunger and satiety cues rather than using controlling feeding practices are more likely to have children with healthy weight outcomes.

•      Avoidance of Restriction: Restrictive feeding practices, such as restricting certain foods, may be associated with an increased risk of overeating and obesity later in childhood.

4.      Feeding in Response to Emotional Cues:

•      Emotional Eating Habits: Using food as a comfort measure or reward can contribute to emotional eating habits, potentially impacting weight regulation.

•      Long-Term Implications: Children who learn to use food to cope with emotions may be at an increased risk of developing unhealthy eating patterns and obesity in the future.

5.    Parental Modeling of Healthy Eating:

•    Role Modeling: Parents who model healthy eating behaviors are more likely to have children who adopt similar habits.

•    Diverse and Nutrient-Rich Diets: Exposure to diverse, nutrient-rich foods through parental modeling contributes to a positive food environment and healthy eating habits.

6.    Infant Sleep and Nighttime Feeding:

•    Sleep Duration: Disrupted sleep patterns and inadequate sleep duration in infancy have been associated with an increased risk of obesity.

•    Nighttime Feeding Practices: Prolonged nighttime feeding practices may disrupt sleep patterns and potentially contribute to an increased risk of obesity.

7.    Responsive Feeding to Hunger and Fullness:

•    Teaching Self-Regulation: Encouraging children to listen to their hunger and fullness cues promotes self-regulation and may contribute to a lower risk of overeating.

•    Avoidance of Forced Eating: Forcing children to finish meals or consume specific amounts may interfere with their ability to self-regulate and impact weight outcomes.

8.    Introduction to Sugar-Sweetened Beverages:

•    Early Exposure: Early introduction to sugar-sweetened beverages may contribute to increased caloric intake and a higher risk of obesity.

• Water as a Primary Beverage: Encouraging water as the primary beverage helps establish healthy hydration habits and reduces the consumption of sugary drinks.

9. Nutritional Quality of Early Diet:

• Diverse Nutrient Sources: Providing a variety of nutrient-rich foods supports optimal growth and development, reducing the risk of nutritional deficiencies.

• Balanced Macronutrient Intake: Ensuring a balanced intake of proteins, fats, and carbohydrates helps establish healthy eating patterns.

10. Parental Education and Support:

• Nutritional Knowledge: Parents with a good understanding of nutrition are better equipped to make informed feeding decisions that support healthy growth.

•      Community Support: Access to community resources and support networks enhances parental capacity to provide a nourishing and supportive feeding environment.

Promoting positive early feeding practices involves a holistic approach that considers both nutritional and psychosocial factors. Providing support, education, and resources for parents and caregivers can empower them to create a nurturing feeding environment that fosters healthy eating habits and reduces the risk of childhood obesity.

❖ **Childhood Obesity and Its Long-Term Consequences:**

Childhood obesity is a complex health issue with far-reaching consequences that extend into adulthood. Understanding the long-term implications of childhood obesity is crucial for public health interventions and the development of strategies to prevent and manage this condition. Here are the significant long-term consequences associated with childhood obesity:

1.    Increased Risk of Adult Obesity:

•    Persistence into Adulthood: Children with obesity are more likely to carry excess weight into adulthood, leading to a higher risk of obesity-related complications later in life.

•    Continued Health Challenges: Long-term adult obesity is associated with an increased risk of chronic diseases, including cardiovascular diseases, diabetes, and certain cancers.

2.    Cardiovascular Health Issues:

•    Atherosclerosis: Childhood obesity contributes to the development of atherosclerosis, the hardening and narrowing of arteries, increasing the risk of heart disease in adulthood.

•    Hypertension: Obese children are more likely to develop hypertension, and this risk often persists into adulthood, contributing to cardiovascular problems.

3.    Type 2 Diabetes:

•    Insulin Resistance: Childhood obesity is a significant risk factor for insulin resistance, a precursor to type 2 diabetes.

•    Early Onset: Children with obesity face an increased likelihood of developing type 2 diabetes at an earlier age, leading to a longer duration of the condition and associated complications.

4.    Metabolic Syndrome:

•    Cluster of Risk Factors: Childhood obesity is linked to the development of metabolic syndrome, characterized by a cluster of risk factors, including high blood pressure, abnormal lipid levels, insulin resistance, and abdominal obesity.

•	Prolonged Health Consequences: Metabolic syndrome increases the risk of cardiovascular diseases and type 2 diabetes in adulthood.

5.	Orthopedic Issues:

•	Musculoskeletal Strain: Excess body weight in childhood places additional stress on the musculoskeletal system, leading to orthopedic issues such as joint pain, arthritis, and an increased risk of fractures.

•	Long-Term Mobility Impairments: Obesity-related orthopedic problems may persist into adulthood, affecting mobility and overall quality of life.

6.	Psychosocial and Mental Health Impact:

•      Low Self-Esteem and Stigmatization: Childhood obesity is often associated with low self-esteem, stigmatization, and poor body image, which may persist into adulthood.

•      Mental Health Disorders: The psychosocial impact can contribute to the development of mental health disorders, including depression and anxiety, with long-term implications for overall well-being.

7.     Liver Disease:

•      Non-Alcoholic Fatty Liver Disease (NAFLD): Childhood obesity is a significant risk factor for NAFLD, which may progress to more severe liver conditions, such as non-alcoholic steatohepatitis (NASH) and cirrhosis, in adulthood.

8.     Respiratory Complications:

• Obstructive Sleep Apnea: Childhood obesity is associated with an increased risk of obstructive sleep apnea, a condition that can persist into adulthood and contribute to respiratory complications.

• Asthma: Obesity is a risk factor for the development and exacerbation of asthma, leading to long-term respiratory challenges.

9. Increased Cancer Risk:

• Association with Certain Cancers: Childhood obesity is linked to an increased risk of developing certain cancers in adulthood, including breast, colorectal, and endometrial cancers.

10. Social and Economic Impact:

• Reduced Educational Attainment: Childhood obesity may be associated with lower educational attainment, potentially impacting future employment opportunities and economic outcomes.

•       Healthcare Costs: The long-term health consequences of childhood obesity contribute to increased healthcare costs, both for individuals and society as a whole.

Addressing childhood obesity requires comprehensive efforts involving healthcare providers, educators, policymakers, and communities. Early prevention and intervention strategies, focusing on promoting healthy lifestyles and creating supportive environments, are essential for mitigating the long-term consequences associated with childhood obesity and improving overall population health.

❖ **Parental Influence on Children's Eating Habits and Physical Activity:**

Parents play a pivotal role in shaping the lifestyle choices, including eating habits and physical activity, of their children. The environment created at home, parental behaviors, and the examples set by parents significantly influence a child's health and well-being. Understanding the impact of parental influence is crucial for promoting healthy behaviors in children. Here's an exploration of how parents influence their children's eating habits and physical activity:

1.    Role Modeling:

•    Observational Learning: Children learn by observing and imitating their parents. Parents who model healthy eating habits and an active lifestyle set a positive example for their children to follow.

•    Behavioral Imitation: Children are more likely to adopt eating patterns and physical activity levels similar to those of their parents, emphasizing the importance of positive role modeling.

2.    Food Choices and Availability:

•    Home Food Environment: Parents shape the food environment at home by making decisions about the types of foods available. Offering a variety of nutritious foods and limiting the availability of unhealthy snacks fosters healthy eating habits.

•    Meal Planning and Preparation: Involving children in meal planning and preparation can increase their awareness of nutritious food choices and encourage a positive relationship with food.

3.    Feeding Practices:

•    Responsive Feeding: Parents who respond to their child's hunger and satiety cues, allowing the child to regulate their own food intake, contribute to the development of healthy eating habits.

• Avoidance of Restriction: Restrictive feeding practices, such as forbidding certain foods, may lead to increased interest in and overconsumption of restricted foods.

4. Encouraging Healthy Snacking:

• Availability of Snack Options: Parents influence children's snacking habits by providing a selection of healthy snack options, such as fruits, vegetables, and nuts.

• Establishing Snacking Patterns: Encouraging structured and balanced snacking can contribute to better overall nutrition.

5. Mealtime Environment:

• Positive Mealtime Atmosphere: Creating a positive and relaxed mealtime environment fosters healthy associations with food. Family meals provide an opportunity for connection and shared experiences.

•      Encouraging Communication: Open communication during meals allows parents to educate children about nutrition and engage in conversations about healthy choices.

6.     Physical Activity as Family Time:

•      Family Exercise Routine: Parents can make physical activity enjoyable by involving the whole family in activities such as walks, bike rides, or sports.

•      Modeling Active Lifestyles: Parents who prioritize and participate in physical activity demonstrate its importance and positively influence their children's attitudes toward exercise.

7.     Limiting Screen Time:

- Setting Screen Time Limits: Parents play a crucial role in establishing and enforcing guidelines for screen time, encouraging children to engage in more physically active pursuits.

- Screen-Free Family Time: Allocating specific times for screen-free family activities promotes physical activity and reduces sedentary behaviors.

8. Educational Conversations:

- Nutritional Education: Parents can educate their children about the nutritional value of foods, helping them make informed choices.

- Promoting Awareness: Discussing the importance of a balanced diet and regular physical activity fosters awareness and empowers children to make healthy decisions.

9.   Encouraging Outdoor Play:

•     Providing Outdoor Opportunities: Parents who facilitate and encourage outdoor play contribute to children's physical development, coordination, and overall well-being.

•     Active Family Outings: Choosing activities that involve physical movement, such as hiking or playing sports together, promotes a family culture of active living.

10.  Positive Reinforcement:

•     Celebrating Healthy Choices: Reinforcing and celebrating healthy eating habits and active behaviors with positive reinforcement can motivate children to continue making positive choices.

•     Fostering a Positive Body Image: Encouraging a positive body image and emphasizing the importance of overall well-being over appearance contributes to a healthy mindset.

11.   Creating Healthy Habits Early:

•       Establishing Routines: Consistent routines for meals, snacks, and physical activity help children develop healthy habits that can persist into adolescence and adulthood.

•       Long-Term Impact: Early exposure to positive influences from parents can contribute to a lifetime of healthy behaviors.

Recognizing the influential role of parents in shaping children's eating habits and physical activity underscores the importance of family-based interventions for promoting a healthy lifestyle. Empowering parents with knowledge, resources, and support can enhance their ability to positively influence their children's well-being and set the stage for lifelong health.

# CHAPTER 10: PREVENTION AND INTERVENTION STRATEGIES FOR CHILDHOOD OBESITY

Preventing and addressing childhood obesity requires a comprehensive and multi-faceted approach that involves families, communities, schools, and healthcare systems. Implementing effective strategies early in life can significantly reduce the risk of obesity-related complications. Here are key prevention and intervention strategies:

1.    Promoting Healthy Eating Habits:

•    Nutrition Education: Implement school-based and community programs that educate children and parents about the importance of balanced nutrition, understanding food labels, and making healthy food choices.

•	School Meal Programs: Ensure that school meals meet nutritional guidelines and provide access to a variety of nutrient-rich foods.

2.	Encouraging Regular Physical Activity:

•	Physical Education in Schools: Incorporate regular and structured physical education classes in schools to ensure that children engage in age-appropriate physical activities.

•	Recess and Active Breaks: Promote active breaks and recess periods to encourage children to engage in play and physical movement during the school day.

3.	Limiting Screen Time:

•	Educating on Screen Time Guidelines: Provide guidelines to parents on limiting screen time for children, emphasizing the importance of outdoor play and other physically active pursuits.

• Creating Screen-Free Zones: Designate specific areas in homes as screen-free zones to encourage alternative activities like reading, playing, or outdoor recreation.

4. Family-Based Interventions:

• Parental Involvement: Engage parents in educational programs that focus on nutrition, cooking skills, and the importance of physical activity for the entire family.

• Family Wellness Initiatives: Implement family-oriented wellness initiatives that include healthy cooking classes, group activities, and support networks.

5. Community Engagement:

• Community Gardens: Establish community gardens to promote access to fresh, locally grown produce and encourage community involvement in healthy food choices.

• Physical Activity Programs: Develop community-based physical activity programs, such as walking groups, sports leagues, or fitness classes for families.

6. School Wellness Policies:

• Implementing Wellness Policies: Schools should adopt and implement comprehensive wellness policies that address nutrition standards, physical activity, and health education.

• Healthy Celebrations: Encourage schools to promote healthy celebrations, offering nutritious alternatives to traditional sugary snacks and treats.

7. Health Education Programs:

• Early Childhood Education: Integrate health education into early childhood programs to instill healthy habits from an early age.

•      Teen-Specific Education: Tailor health education programs for adolescents, focusing on body image, nutrition, and the importance of regular exercise.

8.    Healthcare Provider Involvement:

•      Regular Well-Child Checkups: Encourage regular well-child checkups where healthcare providers assess growth, development, and nutrition, providing guidance to parents on healthy habits.

•      Screening and Counseling: Incorporate routine obesity screening and counseling during healthcare visits to address potential concerns early and provide necessary support.

9.    Policy Changes:

•	Sugar Reduction Initiatives: Advocate for policies aimed at reducing added sugars in children's diets, including regulations on sugary beverages and snacks.

•	Active Transportation: Support policies that promote active transportation, such as walking or biking to school, to increase physical activity.

10.	Supportive Environments:

•	Safe Play Spaces: Create safe and accessible play spaces in communities to encourage outdoor activities and physical play.

•	Accessible Healthy Foods: Ensure that neighborhoods have easy access to affordable and nutritious food options, reducing reliance on convenience stores with limited healthy choices.

11.	Parental Guidance on Feeding Practices:

•	Responsive Feeding: Encourage parents to adopt responsive feeding practices, allowing children to regulate their own food intake and promoting a healthy relationship with food.

•	Family Meals: Promote regular family meals as an opportunity for connection, communication, and the modeling of healthy eating behaviors.

12.	Collaboration Across Sectors:

•	School-Community Partnerships: Foster collaboration between schools, healthcare providers, community organizations, and policymakers to create a supportive environment for healthy living.

•	Joint Initiatives: Develop joint initiatives that address childhood obesity from multiple angles, including nutrition, physical activity, and community engagement.

Implementing these strategies requires a coordinated effort from various stakeholders, emphasizing education, environmental changes, and supportive policies. By combining these approaches, communities can create an environment that promotes healthy behaviors and reduces the prevalence of childhood obesity.

## ❖ Importance of a Multidimensional Approach in Addressing Childhood Obesity:

A multidimensional approach is crucial for effectively addressing childhood obesity because it recognizes the complexity of the issue and acknowledges that multiple factors contribute to its development. By integrating various strategies across different domains, a multidimensional approach ensures a comprehensive and holistic response. Here's why a multidimensional approach is important:

1.	Complexity of Childhood Obesity:

•	Interconnected Factors: Childhood obesity is influenced by a multitude of interconnected factors, including genetics, environment, socio-economic status, cultural norms, and individual behaviors. A single-dimensional approach may not adequately address this complexity.

2.	Behavioral, Environmental, and Genetic Factors:

•	Behavioral Interventions: Targeting individual behaviors, such as promoting healthy eating and physical activity, is essential. However, considering environmental influences and genetic predispositions ensures a more comprehensive understanding and tailored interventions.

3.    Early Prevention and Intervention:

•    Lifelong Impact: Addressing childhood obesity early is crucial, as habits formed during childhood often persist into adulthood. A multidimensional approach allows for interventions at various stages of a child's development, reducing the risk of long-term health consequences.

4.    Influence of Family and Community:

•    Family Dynamics: Families play a central role in shaping a child's lifestyle. A multidimensional approach recognizes the influence of family dynamics, incorporating interventions that involve parents and caregivers in promoting healthy behaviors.

•    Community Support: Engaging communities in promoting health through accessible resources, safe spaces, and collaborative efforts strengthens the impact of interventions.

5.    Educational and Cultural Sensitivity:

•    Tailored Education: Recognizing diverse educational needs ensures that interventions are culturally sensitive and resonate with various communities. This is crucial for effective communication and engagement.

•    Cultural Competence: Understanding cultural contexts helps tailor interventions to specific communities, considering cultural norms, dietary preferences, and lifestyle practices.

6.    Policy and Environmental Changes:

•    Advocacy for Policy Changes: A multidimensional approach involves advocating for policies that support healthy environments, such as regulating food marketing to children, improving school nutrition standards, and creating walkable neighborhoods.

•	Environmental Modifications: Designing environments that facilitate physical activity, like building parks and sidewalks, contributes to sustained lifestyle changes.

7.	Integration of Healthcare and Public Health:

•	Healthcare Provider Involvement: Integrating healthcare providers into prevention and intervention efforts ensures early identification of potential concerns and the provision of guidance to families.

•	Public Health Initiatives: Public health campaigns, supported by healthcare providers, amplify the impact of interventions by reaching a wider audience and fostering community-wide awareness.

8.	Comprehensive School-Based Programs:

•	Curriculum Integration: Incorporating nutrition education and physical activity into school curricula promotes a culture of health within educational settings.

•	Wellness Policies: Establishing and enforcing comprehensive school wellness policies creates an environment that supports healthy eating and physical activity.

9.	Long-Term Sustainable Changes:

•	Systemic Changes: A multidimensional approach addresses systemic issues, fostering changes in societal norms, food environments, and physical activity infrastructure that contribute to sustained, long-term impact.

•	Behavioral Economics: Incorporating insights from behavioral economics helps design interventions that consider human decision-making, making healthy choices more accessible and appealing.

10.	Preventing Stigmatization:

•	Holistic Health Promotion: A multidimensional approach emphasizes holistic health promotion rather than focusing solely on weight. This reduces the risk of stigmatization and fosters a positive, inclusive environment for children and families.

11.	Collaboration Among Stakeholders:

•	Intersectoral Collaboration: Childhood obesity is a multifaceted challenge that requires collaboration among healthcare professionals, educators, policymakers, community leaders, and families. A multidimensional approach facilitates cooperation among diverse stakeholders.

12.   Tailored Interventions for Various Age Groups:

•      Age-Appropriate Strategies: Different age groups have unique needs and challenges. Tailoring interventions to specific developmental stages ensures that strategies are age-appropriate and resonate with children, adolescents, and their families.

By addressing childhood obesity through a multidimensional lens, interventions become more nuanced, adaptable, and effective. This comprehensive approach recognizes the interplay of various factors, embraces diversity, and ensures that efforts are both inclusive and sustainable for promoting the health and well-being of children and their communities.

## ❖ Public Health Initiatives in Addressing Childhood Obesity:

Public health initiatives are essential components of comprehensive strategies to tackle childhood obesity at a population level. These initiatives aim to create supportive environments, raise awareness, and implement policies that promote healthy lifestyles. Here are key elements of public health initiatives in addressing childhood obesity:

1.    Health Education Campaigns:

•    Nutrition Education: Implement public health campaigns that educate parents, caregivers, and communities about the importance of balanced nutrition, portion control, and making informed food choices.

• Physical Activity Promotion: Develop campaigns that highlight the significance of regular physical activity for children's health and well-being, emphasizing fun and enjoyable activities.

2. School-Based Interventions:

• Comprehensive Wellness Policies: Advocate for and support the implementation of comprehensive school wellness policies that address nutrition standards, physical activity requirements, and health education.

• Healthier School Environments: Work towards creating school environments that prioritize healthy food options in cafeterias, provide opportunities for physical activity, and integrate health education into the curriculum.

3. Community Programs:

•	Community Gardens: Establish and support community gardens to promote access to fresh produce and engage communities in growing their own nutritious foods.

•	Active Living Initiatives: Develop community-wide programs that encourage active living, such as walkability campaigns, community sports leagues, and fitness classes.

4.	Policy Advocacy:

•	Sugar Reduction Policies: Advocate for policies that regulate the marketing and sale of sugary beverages and snacks, with a focus on reducing added sugars in children's diets.

•	School Nutrition Standards: Support and promote policies that establish and enforce nutrition standards in school meals to ensure they align with health guidelines.

5.    Public Spaces and Infrastructure:

•    Safe Play Spaces: Invest in the development of safe and accessible play spaces, parks, and recreational areas that encourage physical activity among children.

•    Active Transportation Planning: Collaborate with urban planners to create neighborhoods that facilitate active transportation, making it easier for families to walk or bike.

6.    Parental Support Programs:

•    Parenting Workshops: Conduct workshops and programs that provide parents with information and skills to support healthy eating habits, positive feeding practices, and the promotion of physical activity.

•    Family-Based Challenges: Organize family-based challenges and events that encourage joint participation in healthy activities, fostering a sense of community and support.

7.    Media and Advertising Regulation:

•    Restricting Unhealthy Food Marketing: Advocate for regulations that restrict the marketing of unhealthy foods and beverages to children through various media channels.

•    Promoting Positive Messaging: Encourage positive messaging in media that emphasizes healthy behaviors, body positivity, and the importance of overall well-being.

8.    Screen Time Guidelines:

•    Public Awareness Campaigns: Launch public awareness campaigns to educate parents and caregivers about recommended screen time limits for children, promoting alternative activities that support physical and mental health.

•	Digital Literacy Programs: Develop digital literacy programs that empower families to make informed decisions about screen time and technology use.

9.	Healthcare Integration:

•	Routine Obesity Screening: Integrate routine obesity screening during well-child checkups to identify potential concerns early and provide timely guidance to parents.

•	Referral Systems: Establish referral systems that connect families with community resources, nutritionists, and physical activity programs to support healthy lifestyles.

10.	Evaluation and Research:

•	Monitoring and Evaluation: Implement ongoing monitoring and evaluation systems to assess the effectiveness of public health initiatives in reducing childhood obesity rates.

•      Research on Best Practices: Invest in research to identify and promote best practices in public health interventions, ensuring evidence-based strategies guide future initiatives.

11.   Collaborative Partnerships:

•      Intersectoral Collaboration: Collaborate with schools, healthcare providers, community organizations, local businesses, and policymakers to create a cohesive and coordinated effort in addressing childhood obesity.

•      Shared Resources: Pool resources and expertise from various sectors to maximize the impact of public health initiatives and create synergies in addressing the complex issue of childhood obesity.

Public health initiatives are instrumental in creating a supportive environment that empowers individuals and communities to make healthier choices.

By combining education, policy advocacy, community engagement, and evaluation, these initiatives contribute to a holistic approach that addresses the multifaceted nature of childhood obesity and promotes sustainable change at both individual and population levels.

❖ **Individual Responsibility and Lifestyle Modifications in Addressing Childhood Obesity:**

While public health initiatives and environmental changes play a crucial role, individual responsibility and lifestyle modifications are equally important in the effort to combat childhood obesity. Empowering individuals, particularly parents and children, to make healthier choices fosters a sense of ownership over one's health. Here are key aspects of individual responsibility and lifestyle modifications in addressing childhood obesity:

1.    Nutrition Education and Meal Planning:

•     Parental Education: Provide parents with resources and information on balanced nutrition, helping them make informed decisions about their children's diets.

•     Meal Planning Skills: Equip families with practical skills for meal planning, preparation, and cooking nutritious meals at home.

2.    Portion Control and Mindful Eating:

•     Teaching Portion Awareness: Educate both parents and children about appropriate portion sizes to avoid overeating.

•     Mindful Eating Practices: Encourage mindful eating, emphasizing the importance of paying attention to hunger and fullness cues.

3.    Healthy Snacking Habits:

•    Promoting Nutrient-Rich Snacks: Encourage the consumption of healthy snacks, such as fruits, vegetables, and nuts, while minimizing the intake of sugary and processed snacks.

•    Limiting Frequency of Snacking: Advocate for balanced and structured snacking, avoiding excessive snacking between meals.

4.    Increased Physical Activity:

•    Family-Based Activities: Promote physical activities that families can engage in together, such as walks, bike rides, or organized sports.

•    Incorporating Play into Daily Life: Encourage unstructured playtime for children, both indoors and outdoors, to increase overall physical activity levels.

5.  Screen Time Management:

•  Setting Screen Time Limits: Establish and enforce guidelines for screen time, encouraging alternative activities that involve movement and social interaction.

•  Educating on Balanced Technology Use: Teach children about the importance of balancing screen time with other activities for overall well-being.

6.  Hydration Habits:

•  Promoting Water Consumption: Emphasize the importance of water as the primary beverage, reducing the intake of sugary drinks.

•  Hydration Awareness: Educate parents and children about the benefits of staying hydrated and recognizing thirst cues.

7.  Sleep Hygiene:

•	Establishing Bedtime Routines: Support the establishment of consistent bedtime routines to ensure adequate and quality sleep for children.

•	Limiting Electronic Device Use Before Bed: Encourage the reduction of screen time, particularly electronic device use, before bedtime to promote better sleep.

8.	Encouraging Outdoor Play:

•	Creating Playful Environments: Foster environments that encourage outdoor play, with access to parks, playgrounds, and open spaces.

•	Active Family Outings: Plan family outings that involve physical activities, such as hiking, biking, or playing sports together.

9.	Behavioral Strategies for Healthy Eating:

•	Positive Reinforcement: Reinforce healthy eating behaviors with positive reinforcement, acknowledging and celebrating good choices.

•	Gradual Changes: Advocate for small, gradual changes in dietary habits, making it easier for individuals to adopt and sustain healthier practices.

10.	Parental Modeling:

•	Leading by Example: Parents who model healthy behaviors, both in terms of nutrition and physical activity, have a significant impact on shaping their children's habits.

•	Open Communication: Create an environment where open communication about health and well-being is encouraged, fostering a positive relationship with food and body image.

11.	Goal Setting and Tracking Progress:

•      Setting Realistic Goals: Encourage families to set realistic and achievable health goals, considering their unique circumstances and preferences.

•      Tracking Progress: Implement tracking mechanisms, such as food diaries or activity logs, to monitor progress and identify areas for improvement.

12.   Promoting Body Positivity:

•      Positive Body Image Messages: Promote positive body image messages to children, emphasizing the importance of health and well-being over unrealistic body ideals.

•      Encouraging Self-Esteem: Foster a supportive environment that encourages children to develop a positive self-image and self-esteem.

Individual responsibility and lifestyle modifications are integral components of a comprehensive approach to childhood obesity. By empowering individuals to make healthier choices and adopt sustainable lifestyle habits, the collective impact can contribute to long-term positive health outcomes for both children and their families.

# CHAPTER 11: CONCLUSION

In conclusion, addressing childhood obesity is a multifaceted challenge that demands a comprehensive and coordinated response from individuals, families, communities, and policymakers. The intricate interplay of genetic, environmental, behavioral, and societal factors underscores the necessity of a multidimensional approach. This comprehensive strategy involves public health initiatives, individual responsibility, and lifestyle modifications to create an environment that promotes healthy living.

Public health initiatives play a pivotal role in shaping policies, raising awareness, and fostering supportive environments. These initiatives target schools, communities, and media, aiming to instill healthy behaviors, regulate marketing practices, and provide resources for families. By advocating for policy changes, creating accessible play spaces, and implementing educational campaigns, public health initiatives contribute to the prevention and reduction of childhood obesity on a population level.

Simultaneously, individual responsibility and lifestyle modifications are crucial components of the solution. Empowering individuals, especially parents and children, to make informed choices regarding nutrition, physical activity, and overall well-being is essential. By promoting healthy eating habits, encouraging regular physical activity, managing screen time, and fostering positive body image, individuals can take ownership of their health and contribute to long-term lifestyle changes.

The integration of both public health initiatives and individual efforts creates a synergistic approach that addresses childhood obesity comprehensively. This collaborative strategy acknowledges the diversity of factors contributing to obesity, from genetic predispositions to societal influences, and seeks to create lasting changes at various levels of society. The importance of early prevention, education, and supportive environments cannot be overstated, as habits formed during childhood often shape lifelong behaviors.

In the pursuit of a healthier future for our children, it is crucial to continue advancing research, refining strategies, and fostering collaboration among stakeholders. By working together to implement evidence-based interventions, promote positive societal attitudes, and empower individuals to lead healthier lives, we can strive towards a world where childhood obesity is minimized, and the well-being of every child is prioritized. Ultimately, the collective efforts of communities, healthcare providers, policymakers, and individuals will pave the way for a healthier and brighter future for the generations to come.

❖ **Recap of Major Causes of Obesity:**

In this comprehensive exploration of the causes of obesity, various factors contribute to the complex nature of this global health concern. Here's a recap of the major causes discussed:

I. Genetic Factors:

•      Role of Genetics: Genetic predispositions play a significant role in influencing an individual's susceptibility to obesity.

•      Family History: Family history is a key factor, with a genetic link influencing the likelihood of obesity within families.

•    Genetic Conditions: Certain genetic conditions contribute to weight gain and obesity, emphasizing the impact of genetic factors on metabolism.

II. Environmental Factors:

•    Influence of the Obesogenic Environment: Modern environments contribute to an obesogenic setting, where factors promote overeating and sedentary behaviors.

•    Availability of High-Calorie Foods: The easy availability and accessibility of high-calorie, processed foods contribute to unhealthy dietary habits.

•    Sedentary Lifestyle: Increased screen time, sedentary jobs, and reduced physical activity contribute to the prevalence of obesity.

III. Behavioral Factors:

•    Dietary Habits and Choices: Unhealthy dietary habits, including the consumption of high-calorie, low-nutrient foods, contribute to excess calorie intake.

•      Physical Activity: Insufficient physical activity, coupled with sedentary lifestyles, contributes to an energy imbalance and weight gain.

IV. Socioeconomic Factors:

•      Economic Disparities: Disparities in economic status influence access to healthy food options and opportunities for physical activity.

•      Access to Health Care: Limited access to healthcare resources may impact preventive measures and obesity management.

•      Education and Awareness: Socioeconomic factors influence education levels and awareness, affecting lifestyle choices and health behaviors.

## V. Psychological Factors:

• Emotional Eating: Emotional factors, such as stress and emotional eating, contribute to unhealthy eating patterns.

• Stress and Eating Behaviors: Chronic stress can lead to changes in eating behaviors, impacting weight management.

• Mental Health Issues: Certain mental health conditions contribute to weight gain and obesity.

## VI. Medical Conditions:

• Hormonal Imbalances: Hormonal factors affecting metabolism can contribute to weight gain and obesity.

• Medications and Medical Conditions: Some medications and certain medical conditions have side effects that may lead to weight gain.

- Impact on Obesity Risk: Underlying medical conditions can increase the risk of obesity.

VII. Cultural and Social Influences:

- Cultural Norms: Cultural attitudes towards body image and food choices influence individual behaviors.

- Social Acceptance of Unhealthy Behaviors: Societal acceptance of unhealthy behaviors may contribute to the normalization of obesity.

- Peer Pressure: Peer influences play a role in shaping lifestyle choices, including diet and physical activity.

VIII. Childhood and Early-life Influences:

- Early Feeding Practices: Early feeding practices and dietary patterns during childhood impact long-term obesity risk.

•      Childhood Obesity Consequences: Childhood obesity has long-term consequences, increasing the risk of adult obesity and associated health issues.

❖ By understanding the interplay of these factors, individuals, healthcare providers, policymakers, and communities can develop targeted interventions and strategies to address the root causes of obesity and work towards effective prevention and management.

## ❖ Call to Action for Addressing the Obesity Epidemic:

The obesity epidemic demands urgent and concerted efforts from individuals, communities, healthcare professionals, policymakers, and society as a whole. A comprehensive call to action is essential to effectively combat this global health crisis. Here are key steps for a collective response:

1.    Promoting Health Education:

•    For Individuals: Emphasize the importance of nutritional literacy and educate individuals on making informed food choices. Encourage understanding of portion control and the significance of balanced diets.

•    For Communities: Implement widespread health education campaigns that reach diverse populations, focusing on schools, workplaces, and community centers.

2.    Encouraging Physical Activity:

•    For Individuals: Advocate for at least 150 minutes of moderate-intensity or 75 minutes of vigorous-intensity physical activity per week. Promote enjoyable and sustainable activities to make exercise a regular part of daily life.

•	For Communities: Develop and support initiatives that create accessible and safe spaces for physical activity. Encourage community events, sports leagues, and fitness programs.

3.	Supporting Policy Changes:

•	For Policymakers: Enact and enforce policies that regulate the marketing and sale of unhealthy foods, especially to children. Implement and strengthen school wellness policies, ensuring nutritious meals and increased physical activity.

•	For Advocates: Advocate for policies that promote walkable neighborhoods, limit sugary beverage consumption, and improve access to healthy foods in underserved communities.

4.     Fostering a Positive Food Environment:

•     For Individuals: Choose nutrient-dense foods over processed, high-calorie options. Embrace a diverse and balanced diet that includes fruits, vegetables, whole grains, and lean proteins.

•     For Retailers: Promote healthier food options and implement transparent labeling in grocery stores. Consider initiatives that incentivize the availability of nutritious foods.

5.     Encouraging Mental Well-being:

•     For Healthcare Providers: Integrate mental health screening into routine care, addressing emotional factors that may contribute to obesity. Collaborate with mental health professionals for comprehensive patient care.

•      For Employers: Create a supportive work environment that prioritizes employee mental health, offering resources and programs to manage stress and promote well-being.

6.     Prioritizing Childhood Health:

•      For Parents and Caregivers: Instill healthy eating habits and an active lifestyle in children from an early age. Limit screen time and prioritize outdoor play.

•      For Schools: Implement comprehensive wellness policies, ensuring nutritious meals, physical education, and health education are integral parts of the curriculum.

7.     Building Supportive Communities:

•      For Community Leaders: Foster a sense of community by organizing events that promote physical activity, healthy eating, and overall well-being.

Collaborate with local organizations to create supportive environments.

•	For Individuals: Engage in community-based initiatives that promote health, creating a network of support for positive lifestyle changes.

8.	Empowering Individuals:

•	For Healthcare Providers: Equip individuals with the knowledge and tools to make informed health choices. Provide resources for goal setting, behavior change, and sustained lifestyle modifications.

•	For Individuals: Take responsibility for personal health by setting realistic goals, seeking support when needed, and making gradual, sustainable changes.

9.	Reducing Stigma and Fostering Inclusivity:

•	For Media and Advertisers: Promote positive body image and portray diverse representations of beauty. Refrain from perpetuating stereotypes that contribute to weight-related stigma.

•	For Schools and Institutions: Implement anti-bullying programs and educate about the importance of inclusivity, ensuring that children and individuals of all sizes feel valued and accepted.

10.	Investing in Research and Innovation:

•	For Researchers: Conduct ongoing research to understand the evolving dynamics of obesity, including genetic, environmental, and behavioral factors. Innovate in the development of effective interventions and treatments.

•	For Funding Agencies: Allocate resources to support obesity research, prevention, and intervention programs. Prioritize initiatives that address health disparities and promote equity.

11.   Collaborating Across Sectors:

•      For Policymakers: Encourage collaboration among healthcare, education, business, and community sectors to develop comprehensive strategies. Leverage the collective strengths of diverse stakeholders to address obesity holistically.

12.   Monitoring and Evaluating Progress:

•      For Governments and Organizations: Establish monitoring and evaluation systems to assess the effectiveness of interventions. Regularly review and adjust strategies based on outcomes to ensure continuous improvement.

By taking collective action and implementing these steps, we can make significant strides in addressing the obesity epidemic. The commitment of individuals, communities, healthcare providers, policymakers, and society at large is essential to create a healthier, more equitable future for generations to come.

❖ **Importance of Ongoing Research and Education in Addressing Obesity:**

Continuous research and education are pivotal components in the multifaceted approach to combat the obesity epidemic. This commitment to advancing knowledge and disseminating information is essential for several reasons:

1.    Understanding Evolving Factors:

• Genetic, Environmental, and Behavioral Dynamics: Ongoing research helps unravel the complex interplay of genetic, environmental, and behavioral factors influencing obesity. Understanding how these factors evolve over time allows for more targeted interventions.

2. Identifying Novel Interventions:

• Innovation in Treatment and Prevention: Research fosters innovation, leading to the identification of novel interventions for both preventing and treating obesity. New insights can inform the development of more effective strategies and therapies.

3. Addressing Health Disparities:

• Tailoring Interventions to Diverse Populations: Research allows for the identification of health disparities related to obesity across different populations. Tailoring interventions based on cultural, socioeconomic, and genetic diversity helps ensure equitable health outcomes.

4.   Monitoring Trends and Patterns:

•   Epidemiological Surveillance: Ongoing research facilitates the monitoring of trends and patterns related to obesity prevalence, allowing for timely interventions and adjustments to public health strategies.

5.   Evaluating Intervention Effectiveness:

•   Continuous Improvement: Research enables the evaluation of the effectiveness of existing interventions. Regular assessments help identify what works, what needs modification, and what can be expanded for broader impact.

6.   Promoting Evidence-Based Practices:

- Guiding Policymakers and Healthcare Providers: Research provides the evidence base for policymakers and healthcare providers to make informed decisions. Evidence-based practices enhance the quality and effectiveness of obesity prevention and management efforts.

7.   Advancing Behavioral Science:

- Behavioral Insights: Ongoing research in behavioral science contributes to a deeper understanding of human behavior related to diet, physical activity, and lifestyle choices. This knowledge is crucial for designing effective behavioral interventions.

8.   Uncovering Underlying Mechanisms:

- Biological and Psychological Mechanisms: Research helps uncover the underlying biological and psychological mechanisms contributing to obesity. This knowledge is fundamental for developing targeted therapies and interventions.

9. Guiding Educational Initiatives:

• Informing Public Health Campaigns: Research findings guide the content and focus of public health campaigns, ensuring that educational initiatives are evidence-based and resonate with diverse populations.

10. Enhancing Medical Training:

• Training Healthcare Professionals: Ongoing education ensures that healthcare professionals are equipped with the latest knowledge and skills for preventing, diagnosing, and managing obesity. This is critical for providing high-quality patient care.

11. Fostering Lifelong Learning:

• Empowering Individuals: Continuous education empowers

individuals to make informed decisions about their health. It promotes a culture of lifelong learning, encouraging individuals to stay updated on nutrition, physical activity, and overall well-being.

12.  Adapting to Societal Changes:

•  Social and Environmental Dynamics: Research helps adapt interventions to societal changes, such as advancements in technology, changes in food environments, and shifts in cultural norms.

In summary, ongoing research and education are the cornerstones of effective obesity prevention and management. By staying at the forefront of scientific knowledge and continuously updating public awareness, we can adapt our strategies to address the ever-evolving challenges posed by obesity. This commitment ensures a dynamic and informed approach to promoting health and well-being for individuals and communities worldwide.

www.ingramcontent.com/pod-product-compliance
Lightning Source LLC
Chambersburg PA
CBHW050801260726
48660CB00004B/1191